Galveston Diet COOKBOOK *for Women over 40*

2000 Days of Hormone-Balancing, Anti-Inflammatory Recipes to Boost Energy & Burn Fat

MONIKA LOVELL

Published by
GRAPEVINE BOOKS

www.grapevinebooks.com
email: contact@grapevinebooks.com

Ordering Information:
Quantity sales: Special discounts are available on quantity purchases by corporations, associations, and others.
For details, reach out to the publisher.

First published by Grapevine Books, 2025

Contents

WELCOME

First things first. If you're reading this, there's a good chance your body has been whispering (or maybe shouting) that something feels different lately. Maybe it's the stubborn belly fat that showed up out of nowhere. Maybe you're exhausted by mid-afternoon, wired at night, or your moods are jumping around like a toddler with a juice box. Maybe you're starting to wonder if it's all in your head or worse, if this is just the "new normal" of getting older.

Let's stop right there. You're not broken. You're not lazy. You're not imagining things. You're in a new phase of life. One that deserves a whole lot more support, clarity, and grace than most of us ever get.

This book was made for you. Not the younger you. Not the you-from-college or the "ideal you" from a Pinterest board. You, right now. The woman who's navigated careers, kids, breakups, marriages, joys, grief, growth, and change. The woman who's been strong for everyone else and is finally ready to turn some of that strength inward.

You don't need another guilt trip. You don't need a trendy cleanse or a short-term fix. You need a framework that's built for real life, real hormones, and real bodies. You need information that makes sense, and food that doesn't feel like a punishment. You need options that feel good in your bones. That's what this book is here for.

You've got wisdom. Now we're giving your body the tools to match.

How This Book Will Change the Way You Eat, Feel, and Live

This isn't a diet book in the traditional sense. It's not about rules. It's about rhythm. You already know that what worked for you in your thirties might not cut it now. That your sleep, weight, mood, and energy are more sensitive than ever. What this book does is help you stop guessing and start understanding what your body is actually asking for.

Here's the reality: hormones matter. They're not just about reproductive stuff. They run the whole show. From the way you burn fat to the way you sleep, from brain fog to bloating, hormones are deeply involved. And in midlife, they don't just change. They throw a party, rearrange the furniture, and then leave you to clean up the mess.

But we're not helpless. With the right habits, you can gently guide those hormonal shifts into something that actually works for you. That's what the Galveston-inspired approach is all about.

Instead of calorie counting or food shaming, we focus on when you eat, what you eat, and how your body reacts to those choices. You'll learn about timed eating (which sounds more intense than it is), anti-inflammatory foods that make your body feel less like a war zone, and the power of fiber, fat, and protein when they're on your side.

You'll also learn that fatigue and brain fog don't mean you're lazy. That bloat isn't just a pasta issue. That your body is wise and trying to communicate. This book is here to help you listen.

What's more, you'll get 100 delicious, simple recipes that nourish you without stress. Meals you can cook after a long day. Snacks that support your goals. Even some feel-good treats that won't wreck your progress.

This is about restoring control. Not through restriction, but through understanding.

You'll go from "Why is this happening?" to "Here's what I can do."

Using This Cookbook for 2000 Days of Wellness

Why 2000 days? Because wellness isn't a 30-day reset or a 6-week bootcamp. It's something you build into your life. One choice at a time, one week at a time, one recipe at a time.

This book is designed to grow with you. Whether you're just starting your journey or already deep in hormone research rabbit holes, you'll find what you need here.

You'll start with a refresh. You'll learn about what your hormones are doing, why inflammation matters more now, and how things like insulin resistance and cortisol spikes can be managed with food and rhythm.

Next, you'll walk through the reset. You'll learn how to use timed eating (aka intermittent fasting) in a gentle, doable way, and how to center your meals around the nutrients your body actually needs.

Then comes the fun part. The food. These recipes aren't just good for you. They taste amazing. They're laid out in categories so you can flip to what you need: breakfasts that energize you, lunches that don't cause a crash, dinners that feel like a hug, snacks that support your metabolism, and even low-sugar treats when you want something sweet without a spiral.

Each one was designed with hormones in mind. They help your body balance itself instead of fighting it.

Best of all, the structure of this book is flexible. Use it daily, weekly, seasonally. If you fall off track, there's no guilt. Just pick a page and start again. That's the power of 2000 days. It's not a sprint. It's a path.

And it's one worth walking. Not because someone told you to. But because you finally decided you deserve it.

> Your body isn't misbehaving. It's *adapting*. Let's give it the support it needs instead of *punishing* it for changing.

You might want to print this and tape it to your fridge. Because that's the kind of mindset shift we're aiming for. Not "I have to eat clean," but "I want to feel good." Not "I blew it today," but "Tomorrow's a new day and I know what helps me." Not "Why is this happening to me?" but "I know what to do when this happens."

It's that shift. From reaction to response. That makes all the difference.

And while we're at it, let's talk about permission. You don't need anyone's permission to put yourself first. To cook meals that support your hormones. To skip social obligations so you can get better sleep. To say no to wine if you know it makes you feel foggy and anxious. You get to decide what serves your body and mind best.

This book isn't going to fix everything in a week. It's not supposed to. What it will do is give you a foundation. A compass. A toolkit. Something to lean on when you're tired, overwhelmed, or just need a reminder that you're not crazy. You're just hormonally human.

Why Women Over 40 Need a Different Plan

By the time you reach midlife, your body is undergoing massive change—even if your calendar doesn't reflect it. You may notice mood swings, brain fog, disrupted sleep, or belly fat that appears out of nowhere. These aren't signs of failure—they're signals. Signals that your hormones are shifting and your body needs a new approach.

This diet provides a nutrition plan that's not just about eating clean. It's about eating smart. It teaches you how to recognize and respond to hormonal clues, how to boost energy naturally, and how to build meals that support weight control without deprivation.

What You Can Expect

Once you apply the tools in this book, you'll notice:

- Improved mental clarity and fewer brain fog episodes
- Reduced cortisol crashes and steadier energy throughout the day
- Fat loss focused on the most stubborn areas, especially belly fat
- Better mood stability, deeper sleep, and fewer fatigue episodes
- The confidence of having a lifestyle plan that supports your female wellness, not just a quick fix

PART ONE: YOUR BODY, REWIRED

CHAPTER 1: WHY EVERYTHING FEELS DIFFERENT NOW

1. The Midlife Hormone Shift

Let's just call it what it is. One day, your body feels like yours. You've got routines that work, food that keeps you steady, maybe a workout that makes you feel strong. Then suddenly, it's like someone swapped out the operating system without your permission.

The sleep that used to come so easily now feels broken. You wake up more often. Your weight starts creeping up, even though you're eating the same (or less). Your jeans fit tighter around the middle. And energy? You need two coffees just to pretend you're awake.

It's not just in your head, and it's definitely not just aging. It's hormonal.

Around your late thirties to early forties, your body starts transitioning toward menopause, beginning with perimenopause. This shift can last years, and it's anything but subtle. What's happening inside is a slow, unpredictable recalibration of your entire hormonal network.

Let's start with estrogen. This is the hormone most people associate with "women's health," and for good reason. Estrogen supports everything from your metabolism and skin elasticity to your brain and bones. When estrogen starts to fluctuate, it doesn't just taper down neatly. It swings. One week you may feel amazing, the next like your entire body turned on you. This fluctuation can cause mood swings, irregular periods, and that sudden bloat you can't explain.

Then there's insulin. It's the hormone that manages your blood sugar. As we age, we often become more insulin-resistant, which means your body doesn't process carbs as smoothly. Even healthy carbs may cause crashes or stubborn weight gain around the belly. That's not because you're doing anything wrong. It's because your hormonal response has changed, and now your body stores more fat instead of burning it.

Now let's bring in cortisol, your stress hormone. In your twenties, you could pull an all-nighter, have wine and fries for dinner, and bounce back. But now, even mild stress seems to throw everything off. Cortisol affects how you sleep, how you digest, how you store fat, and how you recover. When it's too high for too long, your body goes into fight-or-flight mode. Your heart races more easily. You feel wired at bedtime. You hold onto fat around your midsection.

Estrogen is packing her things, insulin's moody, and cortisol is throwing a fit in the kitchen. You're just trying to live in the same house with them.

Here's a question I hear all the time: "Why is it always the belly?"

During this phase, many women notice their body shape shifting. The fat that used to show up in the hips or thighs starts accumulating around the waist instead. There's a physiological reason for this.

As estrogen declines, your body loses a hormone that used to help regulate fat distribution. Without its guidance, fat gets stored where cortisol likes to place it, right around your middle. Add in the insulin resistance we talked about, and your body is more likely to store fat than burn it, even if you're eating well.

And this isn't just about appearance. Visceral fat, the kind that gathers around your organs, can also increase your risk of chronic issues like heart disease and type 2 diabetes. But the good news is, your body can still respond beautifully to change. You're not stuck. You just need to shift strategies.

Beyond the scale and waistline, there's a deeper, quieter frustration. Many women in midlife say things like:

- "I don't feel like myself."
- "I used to be sharp. Now I'm forgetful."
- "My energy is gone."
- "I get hot out of nowhere."

"I feel anxious for no reason."

This isn't just emotional or circumstantial. These are hormonal effects. When estrogen dips, it doesn't just affect your reproductive system. It plays a role in how your brain uses energy, how your body regulates temperature, and how you feel day to day. That's why hot flashes, brain fog, and mood shifts tend to cluster together.

Sleep often becomes fractured too. You may fall asleep fine but wake up at 3 a.m. Your body feels tired but wired. That's cortisol talking again. Your stress response is firing at the wrong time, and your melatonin, the sleep hormone, isn't getting the signals it needs.

All of this makes it incredibly hard to know what's going on. And when you feel foggy, tired, bloated, or heavy, your instinct may be to blame yourself or try to "power through." But that only makes the stress cycle worse. What you actually need is understanding.

You need to know that what you're experiencing is a natural, if frustrating, transition. And you need tools, not pressure, to support your body through it. That's the foundation of everything we'll explore next. From nutrition to timing to lifestyle shifts, we'll begin to untangle this hormonal storm and help you build a path forward that makes sense for this version of you.

2. Understanding Perimenopause and Menopause

Let's break down what's really going on with these terms, because most of us didn't get a proper explanation in school. You probably know about menopause, but the truth is, perimenopause is where all the drama starts.

Perimenopause can begin in your late 30s or early 40s and last for several years. It's the time when your hormones begin to fluctuate wildly. Estrogen doesn't just slowly go down. It zigzags. One day it spikes, the next it drops. That's why symptoms can feel so inconsistent. You might feel great for two weeks, then suddenly have three days where you're irritable, bloated, and exhausted for no apparent reason.

Menopause, on the other hand, is officially marked when you've gone a full 12 months without a period. After that point, hormone levels tend to level off, though they remain much lower than they were in your twenties and thirties.

But here's what no one tells you: these phases affect your entire life. They're not just about your period stopping. They're about how your body functions from head to toe. Your metabolism, digestion, immune system, heart health, skin, and brain are all affected. Hormones are like your body's software. And when the system updates, you need new tools to keep everything running smoothly.

One of the hardest parts of this shift is realizing that the things that used to work for you no longer do. That workout you used to love? Now it leaves you drained. That light dinner you counted on to maintain your weight? Suddenly it's not enough to keep your energy up.

This is where frustration tends to pile up. You feel like you're trying harder, but seeing worse results. That disconnect isn't about willpower. It's biological.

In midlife, your body's stress tolerance changes. Long workouts, low-calorie diets, or inconsistent sleep patterns may backfire. Instead of making you leaner or more energized, they can elevate cortisol, drain your reserves, and make your body cling to fat even harder.

And when your hormones are fluctuating, what your body needs isn't more intensity. It's better alignment.

This means shorter, more focused workouts. More consistent eating windows. Meals that are rich in fat, fiber, and protein, not low-fat, high-carb snack packs that leave you crashing by noon.

Your body is wiser now. It's asking for support, not punishment.

Maybe you've felt isolated or unsure. Maybe your doctor brushed off your concerns or told you that "it's just part of getting older." That's not good enough.

The truth is, millions of women are navigating these exact changes at this very moment, quietly wondering if they're the only ones who feel off. You are far from alone.

That's one of the reasons this book was written. To bring these changes into the light. To give you language for what's happening. To offer a plan that doesn't involve starving yourself or pretending everything's fine when it's not.

This part of life can be powerful, freeing, and full of vitality. But not if we keep trying to treat our 47-year-old bodies like they're 27.

When you understand what's changing, and why, it becomes easier to take action. And when those actions are based on science and self-respect, they stick.

We're going to move forward with exactly that: intention. In the next chapter, you'll learn how nutrition, sleep, and mindset all connect to your hormones. You'll start to see patterns instead of problems, and options instead of obstacles.

And most importantly, you'll start to trust your body again.

3. Let's Stop Blaming Ourselves

Somewhere along the way, many women start to think all these changes are somehow their fault. That they've "let themselves go." That if they could just try harder or eat cleaner or work out more, they'd be back to normal. But here's the thing. Yhere's no going back to the old version of you.

That's not a failure. That's evolution.

You are not a project gone wrong. You are a system in transition. Your body is still working for you, even if it's not behaving the way it used to. It's recalibrating. You're experiencing changes that are as real and biological as puberty was. Only this time, instead of being handed a health class booklet and some awkward charts, you're expected to figure it out in silence.

So let's say this clearly.

Despite how it might feel some days, your body hasn't given up on you. It hasn't stopped responding. It's just asking for a different language. What worked for your metabolism at 25 might not be what helps at 45. That doesn't mean you're out of options. It means you're being invited to shift strategies.

And here's the beauty of it. When you do shift, the results are often faster and deeper than you'd expect. Once your body feels supported, it starts to show up for you again. The brain fog starts to lift. Your energy steadies out. The bloat goes down. You sleep more soundly.

You just need the right tools, and a bit of patience while they start to work.

One of the most powerful things you can do during this time is to slow down and pay attention. Start noticing what foods make you feel calm and clear, versus which ones leave you groggy or craving more. Pay attention to your energy rhythms. Are you sharp in the morning but crashing by 3 p.m.? Do you wake up anxious even when you've slept enough?

Your hormones speak in sensations. Bloating, cravings, mood dips, or trouble concentrating—all of these are your body's way of asking for adjustment.

This doesn't mean obsessing over every symptom. It just means staying curious. Noticing what changes help you feel better. Tuning in, instead of zoning out.

Because your body isn't a battleground. It's a communication channel. And once you start listening, it has a lot to say.

Let's talk about something big that gets overlooked: permission.

Most of us have been conditioned to believe that prioritizing our needs is selfish. That slowing down or adjusting expectations is weakness. That asking for help, or choosing rest, or changing routines is something we need to earn. But those ideas? They don't serve you here.

Because midlife isn't a time to push harder. It's a time to tune in more. Your body is working harder behind the scenes than ever before. Your hormones are shifting. Your sleep patterns are evolving. Your emotional landscape may feel raw or unfamiliar. That's not laziness. That's biology calling for backup.

So instead of asking, "What should I be doing?" try asking, "What does my body need today?"

Some days that might be a walk outside. Other days it might be a slow morning and a high-protein breakfast. Some weeks you'll be on fire with meal prep, and other weeks you'll just need to get through. The key is not perfection, but consistency in care.

You're not "cheating" if you modify your workouts. You're not "failing" if you say no to things that drain you. You're actually succeeding when you learn to honor this new version of you.

4. How Balanced Are Your Hormones? Take the Midlife Check-In

Not sure whether what you're feeling is "just stress" or something hormonal? This short quiz will help you identify patterns that may point to perimenopause, menopause, or a transitional hormonal phase. Use your score as a guide for deeper conversations with your healthcare provider and to track how lifestyle shifts (like the Galveston Diet) are working for you.

- Instructions:
- For each symptom, rate the level at which it affects your daily life:

None / Mild / Moderate / Severe

1. Nighttime restlessness or difficulty staying asleep

2. Sudden warmth or flushing in your face or body

3. Unexplained feelings of sadness or low mood

4. Decreased sexual desire or drive

5. Achy joints or stiffness when waking or sitting

6. Brain fog, forgetfulness, or slower thinking

7. Disrupted digestion or feeling "off" after meals

8. Mood swings or feeling emotionally unpredictable

9. Vaginal dryness or discomfort during intimacy

10. New facial hair growth or thinning scalp hair

11. Skin dryness or changes in skin texture

12. Unusual fatigue despite adequate sleep

13. Headaches that feel cyclical or hormone-related

14. Increased urination or urgency

15. Anxiety, restlessness, or feeling "on edge"

Scoring:

None = 0 points

Mild = 1 point

Moderate = 2 points

Severe = 3 points

Your Total Score:

0–15: Minimal or early changes. Your hormones may be stable.

16–30: You may be in the early to mid stages of perimenopause.

31+: Symptoms strongly suggest perimenopause or menopause. Consider support options.

5. The Galveston Diet: Designed for Your Now

By the time you reach the end of this chapter, one truth becomes crystal clear: the rules have changed. Your body doesn't behave the way it used to. Your cravings feel different. Your energy comes and goes. Your favorite healthy habits may not deliver results like they once did.

You haven't failed. You've just outgrown the one-size-fits-all health advice that was never built for this stage of life.

This is where the Galveston Diet comes in, not as a diet in the traditional, restrictive sense, but as a strategic, science-backed framework for women over 40. It was created with the specific challenges of perimenopause and menopause in mind. It speaks your body's new language, and it's designed to work with you, not against you.

So what makes it different?

Most diets focus on weight loss through calorie reduction. They push willpower, cut carbs, and count points, often ignoring how food impacts your hormones. The Galveston Diet flips that approach. It starts by asking a more important question:

What does a midlife body actually need to feel better, think clearer, and burn energy efficiently again?

The answer lies in three powerful pillars:

1. Anti-inflammatory eating
2. Timed eating (intermittent fasting)
3. High-quality, hormone-supportive fats

The answer lies in three powerful pillars:

1. Anti-inflammatory eating
2. Timed eating (intermittent fasting)
3. High-quality, hormone-supportive fats

Let's walk through how each of these directly supports the hormone rollercoaster you've just spent this chapter unpacking.

Anti-Inflammatory Eating: Calming the Chaos

You've already learned that chronic inflammation can quietly disrupt everything, from your sleep and digestion to your mood and waistline. It becomes harder to control as estrogen declines, and the foods that once felt harmless may now leave you bloated, foggy, or flat-out exhausted.

The Galveston Diet tackles inflammation head-on by shifting your focus away from highly processed, sugar-laden, and carb-heavy meals and toward nutrient-dense, whole foods.

This includes:

- Bright, colorful vegetables that are rich in antioxidants
- Leafy greens that soothe inflammation and support detox
- Omega-3 fats from fish, nuts, and seeds
- Spices like turmeric and ginger that calm inflammatory responses
- Clean proteins to stabilize blood sugar and support muscle

When you eat this way consistently, your body begins to feel lighter not just on the scale, but in your joints, your mind, and your digestion. Inflammation drops. Hormones stop spiking. You sleep better, think clearer, and experience fewer crashes.

This isn't a list of "good" and "bad" foods. It's a set of tools to help your midlife body feel safe and supported.

Timed Eating: Restoring Insulin and Energy Flow

One of the biggest hormonal disruptions in midlife is insulin resistance. Your body doesn't handle sugar and carbs the way it used to. Even healthy meals can spike blood sugar and trigger fat storage if your insulin response is out of sync.

Enter intermittent fasting, or as it's called in the Galveston Diet, timed eating.

This isn't about skipping meals or starving yourself. It's about giving your body a consistent eating window, often 8 hours a day, and allowing for 16 hours of rest and repair. That break gives your insulin levels time to reset. It also reduces inflammation, supports fat burning, and can help regulate hunger hormones like leptin and ghrelin.

In short, you become more metabolically flexible.

You don't need to start with a strict plan. Even a 12:12 approach (12 hours eating, 12 hours fasting) can help ease blood sugar swings and calm nighttime cravings.

And because the Galveston Diet pairs this with nourishing, satisfying meals, you're not white-knuckling your way through the day. You feel fed, fueled, and focused.

Healthy Fats: Fueling Hormones and Satiety

If you grew up in the low-fat era, it may feel strange to think of fat as a solution, not a problem. But healthy fats are one of the most powerful allies for hormone health, especially during perimenopause and menopause.

Here's why:

- Fat helps build hormones like estrogen and progesterone
- It keeps you full longer, reducing cravings and snacking
- It supports brain health, especially when fog and fatigue hit
- It helps regulate blood sugar and mood swings

The Galveston Diet encourages a shift toward high-quality fats like avocado, olive oil, nuts, seeds, and fatty fish. These don't make you sluggish or gain weight. They actually help unlock stored energy and give your body the building blocks it needs to heal.

When combined with fiber-rich veggies and moderate protein, fat becomes your body's best stabilizer. You feel more grounded, more satisfied, and less like a prisoner to sugar highs and lows.

Why the Galveston Diet Works for You

Here's the most important takeaway: the Galveston Diet wasn't built for the general public. It was built for you.

It's a response to everything you've been feeling in this chapter:

- The fatigue that shows up despite your efforts
- The bloating that doesn't budge
- The cravings that seem to come out of nowhere
- The sleep that refuses to cooperate
- The belly fat that doesn't respond to workouts
- The fog, the anxiety, the loss of rhythm

This way of eating is gentle but powerful. Structured but flexible. Rooted in research but deeply personal. It asks you to stop punishing your body and start partnering with it.

It says: You don't need to diet harder. You need to nourish smarter.

By choosing this approach, you're not just improving symptoms. You're stepping into a new relationship with your body, one built on respect, understanding, and strength.

You're no longer guessing. You're building a foundation.

And in the next chapter, we'll start laying that foundation one step at a time.

6. The Wisdom in Midlife

Here's something you don't hear enough: you've never been more equipped to take control of your health than you are right now.

You have life experience. You've made mistakes and learned from them. You've faced stress, loss, triumph, and transition. You already know that white-knuckling your way through change isn't the answer.

Now is the time to use that wisdom and apply it to your body with grace, curiosity, and compassion.

You don't have to do everything perfectly. You just have to do the right things consistently. The hormone-friendly meals. The intentional movement. The stress relief rituals that actually help. The sleep habits that reset your nervous system. That's where transformation happens.

And that transformation isn't about going back to who you used to be. It's about becoming someone even stronger, someone aligned with who you are now.

The truth is, most of us were never taught how to support our bodies through this stage. We were handed diet tips, given vague advice to "stay active," and told to expect a few hot flashes. No one mentioned insulin resistance. No one explained how estrogen impacts brain function. No one warned us that our go-to meals or favorite routines might suddenly backfire.

That confusion is real. But it's not where your story ends.

What this chapter has shown you is that every frustrating symptom has a reason. There's a hormonal fingerprint behind the changes you've felt. And while that might sound overwhelming, it's actually empowering. Because now you can work with that knowledge. Now you can stop guessing.

The chapters ahead will give you the tools to do just that, with strategies that are built for your phase of life, your metabolism, your hormones, and your goals. Whether your focus is fat loss, energy, mood, or simply feeling like yourself again, you'll learn how to create a rhythm that restores balance.

So here's your new truth: You are not broken. You are not out of time. You are not in decline.

You are learning a new language, one your body has been trying to speak for a while. And the more fluent you become in that language, the more your daily choices will feel supportive instead of stressful.

Your kitchen becomes a source of energy, not guilt. Your habits become a form of self-trust, not punishment. Your body becomes a partner, not a problem.

This isn't about chasing a younger version of you. This is about stepping into a wiser one.

> This chapter is not the end of who you were. It's the beginning of how strong, capable, and clear you can feel again, with tools made for this chapter of life.

You've taken the first step by reading this far. You've said yes to understanding. Yes to clarity. Yes to healing from the inside out.

Now let's build your foundation.

CHAPTER 2: THE HORMONE AND HEALTH CONNECTION

You've probably heard this before: "You are what you eat." But during midlife, it's more accurate to say, "You feel what you eat."

Because once your hormones start shifting, food stops being just about calories and starts being about chemistry. Every bite you take either supports your hormonal balance or adds to the chaos. And that's not meant to scare you. It's meant to give you power.

The things you eat now have a more immediate impact than they used to. A sugary breakfast might give you brain fog for the rest of the day. A high-carb lunch might lead to a 3 p.m. crash that feels like you've hit a wall. On the flip side, a high-protein breakfast can keep your cravings in check. A fiber-rich lunch can stabilize your blood sugar and give you steady energy into the evening.

Your body is more responsive now. Which means your choices can be more effective too.

This chapter is about helping you understand what those choices are and how they connect to your mood, metabolism, memory, and more.

1. Understanding the Hormonal Web of Perimenopause

Perimenopause is often described as a hormonal transition, but that phrase doesn't quite capture the complexity, or the intensity, of what's actually happening inside the body. During this time, a delicate network of hormones that once worked in relative harmony begins to shift, fluctuate, and, in some cases, decline. These changes don't just affect the reproductive system. They ripple through every major process in the body, from metabolism and mood to digestion, appetite, energy, and even sleep.

While estrogen and progesterone are often named as the "main characters" of this phase, the truth is that a wide array of hormones are involved. The body is a tightly interconnected system. When one hormone shifts, others respond. Some rise to compensate. Others retreat. Some become more dominant than they should. And some, like insulin or cortisol, become more sensitive, amplifying symptoms that can feel confusing or overwhelming.

Understanding how these hormones function individually and together gives women clarity. It explains why fatigue might show up even with adequate rest, why belly fat seems to stick despite regular workouts, and why cravings or anxiety may spike out of nowhere. Knowledge about these hormones turns confusion into confidence and empowers women to make informed choices about how they eat, move, rest, and live during this pivotal phase.

Let's walk through the key hormonal players that influence the perimenopausal journey, starting with the most well-known and progressing into those that, while less talked about, play equally crucial roles in how women feel day to day.

Estrogen shifts affect mood and metabolism, causing unpredictability.
Insulin regulates blood sugar, but resistance increases weight and cravings.
Leptin should signal fullness, but resistance creates constant hunger confusion.
Ghrelin drives appetite, often elevated by stress and poor sleep habits.
Cortisol responds to stress, but chronic spikes disrupt sleep and fat storage.
Neuropeptide Y increases cravings, especially under stress and sleep deprivation.
GLP-1 controls blood sugar and appetite, but declines impair hunger signals.
CCK triggers fullness early. Its imbalance increases overeating.
PYY maintains post-meal fullness, but low levels cause quick return hunger.
Melatonin promotes restful sleep, but disruptions worsen fatigue and cravings.

1. Estrogen: The Master Communicator

Estrogen is the hormone most closely associated with womanhood, and for good reason. It plays a foundational role in reproductive health, yes, but it also impacts the brain, bones, heart, skin, muscles, and metabolism. During perimenopause, estrogen becomes erratic. It doesn't simply decline in a straight line. Instead, it fluctuates dramatically, sometimes surging high and then plummeting low without much warning. These swings are what give rise to many of the classic perimenopausal symptoms.

When estrogen is too low, it can lead to hot flashes, vaginal dryness, night sweats, mood swings, and memory lapses. When it spikes too high (often due to imbalances with progesterone), it can cause breast tenderness, irritability, bloating, and heavy periods. It's this inconsistent behavior, rather than the eventual drop, that tends to create the most chaos in midlife.

Estrogen also directly influences serotonin, the neurotransmitter responsible for feelings of happiness and well-being. This is why emotional changes during perimenopause, like sadness, anxiety, or rage, aren't just psychological. They're biological. When estrogen dips, serotonin availability drops too, leaving you more vulnerable to mood swings.

Another lesser-known effect of estrogen is its impact on insulin sensitivity. Estrogen helps regulate how efficiently your body uses insulin to process glucose. As estrogen decreases, insulin resistance can creep in, making it harder to lose weight and easier to store fat especially around the midsection.

> In short, estrogen is like the *orchestra conductor* of your hormones. When she's erratic or absent, the entire symphony feels *off-key*.

Estrogen also affects bone density, helping maintain the balance between bone breakdown and rebuilding. This is why postmenopausal women are at a higher risk of osteoporosis.

Supporting estrogen balance through diet, stress management, and, for some, hormone therapy can help reduce the turbulence and restore a sense of rhythm to your body.

2. Insulin: The Fat Storage Switch

Insulin is a hormone produced by the pancreas that helps regulate blood sugar levels. It acts like a key, allowing glucose from the bloodstream to enter cells where it can be used for energy. But insulin does much more than manage sugar. It plays a central role in fat storage, hunger, cravings, and even inflammation, all of which become more challenging during perimenopause.

As estrogen begins to fluctuate and decline, insulin sensitivity decreases. This means your cells don't respond as efficiently to insulin's signals. The result? Your body releases more insulin to try to get the job done. This hyperinsulinemia, or elevated insulin, can cause a cascade of problems. It promotes fat storage, particularly around the belly. It triggers more frequent hunger signals. It leads to blood sugar spikes and crashes, which in turn cause cravings for carbs and sugar. Over time, this can contribute to insulin resistance, a condition that dramatically increases the risk for type 2 diabetes, heart disease, and weight gain.

And here's the kicker: even healthy carbs, like brown rice or fruit, can create these spikes in someone with insulin resistance. This is why many women in midlife feel like they gain weight despite eating "clean." Their bodies simply aren't metabolizing nutrients the way they used to.

Insulin is also tied to inflammation, especially when chronically elevated. Inflammatory markers rise, and fat cells, particularly visceral fat, release cytokines that worsen hormonal imbalance and increase disease risk.

Managing insulin in perimenopause means embracing a new nutritional rhythm. Timed eating or intermittent fasting can give insulin levels a break. Pairing carbohydrates with protein and fat helps slow glucose absorption. Prioritizing fiber-rich foods, avoiding ultra-processed snacks, and managing stress all help restore insulin function.

Ultimately, insulin is not the villain. It's just responding to the hormonal chaos around it. When understood and supported, insulin can shift from a fat-storage trigger back into a powerful tool for energy, vitality, and metabolic health.

3. Leptin: The Satiety Signal and Silent Struggler

Leptin, often called the "satiety hormone," plays a crucial role in regulating appetite and metabolism. Produced primarily by fat cells, leptin's main job is to tell your brain, "We've got enough fuel stored. You can stop eating now." It acts as a communication bridge between your body's energy reserves and your hunger response.

In a younger, hormonally balanced body, this system works fairly well. When your fat stores are adequate, leptin rises and curbs appetite. When fat levels drop, leptin falls and stimulates hunger to restore balance. But in perimenopause, this system begins to short-circuit.

As estrogen levels start to fluctuate, leptin signaling becomes less reliable. Even if your body is producing enough leptin, your brain may not get the message. This condition is known as leptin resistance, and it's incredibly common in women entering midlife. In leptin resistance, leptin levels remain high, but the brain becomes desensitized to its signal. Your body acts like it's starving, even if you're not.

The result? You feel hungrier more often, find it harder to feel satisfied after meals, and experience increased cravings, especially in the evening. This mismatch between actual energy stores and perceived hunger leads many women to overeat, often in confusion or frustration. You may wonder, "Why am I still hungry after eating a full meal?" or "Why am I thinking about food even when I'm not physically hungry?"

Sleep disruption plays a major role here too. Leptin levels are partially regulated by the sleep-wake cycle. When sleep is shortened or fragmented, which is common in perimenopause due to night sweats, anxiety, or early waking, leptin levels fall, and your body responds with increased hunger the next day. Compounding the issue, poor sleep also raises ghrelin, the hunger hormone, leading to a double whammy of low satiety and high appetite.

Supporting leptin during perimenopause means working from multiple angles:

- Nourish consistently with whole foods that are rich in protein, fiber, and healthy fat. Crash diets or extreme calorie cuts can reduce leptin production and worsen resistance.

- Get high-quality sleep, ideally 7–9 hours per night. This helps restore hormonal balance and improves leptin sensitivity.

- Move your body regularly, especially with strength training and low-impact cardio. Exercise improves leptin sensitivity and lowers systemic inflammation.

- Manage stress, which interferes with hormonal signaling across the board and worsens metabolic health.

Leptin is not something you feel directly, like a mood or sensation. It works silently in the background, shaping your hunger cues and energy balance. But when it's out of sync, it can make you feel like you've lost control of your appetite. Understanding leptin's role gives you the power to restore that control, not through restriction, but through support and strategy.

4. Ghrelin: The Hunger Hormone You Can't Ignore

While leptin tells your brain to stop eating, ghrelin does the exact opposite. Known as the "hunger hormone," ghrelin is produced in the stomach and signals to the brain when it's time to eat. It rises before meals, creating that familiar gnawing sensation in your belly, and drops after you've eaten.

In a healthy system, ghrelin and leptin work in balance, ghrelin says "go," leptin says "stop." But in perimenopause, this balance often breaks down.

Ghrelin levels can become elevated or erratic, and your body becomes more sensitive to its signal. This is partly due to lower estrogen levels, which seem to reduce the regulation of ghrelin. As a result, you may feel hungrier more often or crave food shortly after meals. And it's not just any food you crave. It's typically quick, high-carb, dopamine-releasing options like bread, chips, sugar, or pastries.

One of the biggest drivers of ghrelin dysregulation is poor sleep. Studies show that even one night of reduced or fragmented sleep can increase ghrelin levels the next day, leading to a measurable rise in appetite, particularly for high-calorie foods. For women navigating night sweats, restless sleep, or anxiety-driven insomnia, this sets up a vicious cycle: less sleep leads to more ghrelin, which leads to overeating, which leads to disrupted digestion and worse sleep.

Ghrelin is also influenced by blood sugar fluctuations. A diet high in refined carbohydrates and low in protein causes quick rises and falls in blood glucose, which can lead to more frequent ghrelin surges. This explains why many women feel ravenous just an hour or two after eating a bowl of cereal or toast, even if the portion was large.

Emotionally, ghrelin interacts with the brain's reward centers. Eating when ghrelin is high triggers a bigger dopamine release, creating a strong emotional feedback loop between hunger and pleasure. This is one reason emotional eating is harder to manage during perimenopause.

To bring ghrelin back into balance, consider the following strategies:

- Prioritize protein at every meal. Protein is more effective than carbs or fat at suppressing ghrelin. Aim for 20–30 grams per meal.

- Eat regular meals, ideally every 4–5 hours. Skipping meals or grazing all day can confuse ghrelin rhythms and lead to excessive hunger spikes.
- Improve your sleep hygiene, focusing on a cool, dark room, screen-free wind-down time, and a consistent bedtime.
- Engage in mindful eating. Slowing down your meals and focusing on satiety can help you recognize when hunger is real versus when it's ghrelin-driven.

In perimenopause, ghrelin is often louder than usual. But that doesn't mean you have to obey every signal. By adjusting your nutrition, stress levels, and sleep habits, you can reduce its intensity and reclaim hunger as something helpful—not overwhelming.

5. Cortisol: The Stress Hormone That Won't Quit

Cortisol is your body's primary stress hormone, produced by the adrenal glands in response to any perceived threat. It plays an essential role in survival: raising blood sugar for energy, improving alertness, and reducing non-essential functions in a crisis. But what happens when the "crisis" is constant and hormonal?

During perimenopause, cortisol levels often become dysregulated. Instead of rising only during short-term stress, cortisol may remain elevated all day or spike at inappropriate times, like 3 a.m. This happens for several reasons. First, as estrogen and progesterone decline, the body loses some of its natural calming, stabilizing signals. Second, perimenopausal symptoms themselves, like poor sleep, mood swings, and hot flashes create more internal stress. Third, many women in midlife are juggling multiple external pressures: aging parents, teenagers, work, relationships, identity shifts.

This results in chronic low-grade cortisol elevation, which quietly undermines health over time. High cortisol contributes to belly fat, especially around the waist, by increasing blood sugar and triggering insulin release. It interferes with sleep, suppresses thyroid function, weakens immune response, and increases inflammation. It can also worsen anxiety, create a sense of urgency or panic, and disrupt mood stability.

Cortisol and estrogen are closely linked. Estrogen helps buffer the body's stress response, but as estrogen drops, cortisol's effects become more pronounced. You may notice that you're more easily startled, more sensitive to noise or conflict, or more prone to snapping under pressure. This isn't just emotional; it's hormonal.

To manage cortisol during perimenopause:

- Prioritize sleep as your top wellness goal. Cortisol can't regulate if rest is poor.
- Exercise wisely. While movement lowers cortisol, too much intensity can backfire. Try walking, Pilates, or yoga.
- Eat for blood sugar stability. Balanced meals with protein, fat, and fiber reduce cortisol spikes caused by glucose crashes.
- Breathe and reset. Even 3 minutes of deep breathing lowers cortisol measurably.
- Carve out calm. Your nervous system needs intentional breaks, like quiet time, nature, laughter, and boundaries.

Cortisol's job is to protect you. But when it overperforms, it can leave you feeling drained, foggy, or "wired but tired." The good news? It responds beautifully to consistent care and nervous system support. You don't have to eliminate stress, just build a better buffer.

6. Neuropeptide Y: The Craving Creator

Neuropeptide Y (NPY) isn't as widely known as cortisol or estrogen, but it plays a major role in how you handle stress, appetite, and energy balance, especially during perimenopause. NPY is a neurotransmitter produced in the brain and sympathetic nervous system. It's one of the most potent appetite stimulators in the body, especially in response to stress.

Here's how it works: when you're under stress, your body releases cortisol and adrenaline to help you cope. That part is expected. But prolonged or repeated stress also leads to the release of NPY, which tells your body to store energy and seek high-calorie food, particularly carbohydrates and fats.

This explains why so many women report strong cravings for comfort foods, like bread, pasta, chips, sweets, when they feel emotionally overwhelmed. It's not weakness. It's your brain chemistry trying to protect you. NPY is essentially preparing the body to survive a famine by increasing appetite and slowing metabolism.

During perimenopause, NPY production becomes more sensitive. Because hormonal fluctuations already create internal stress, your body may overproduce NPY even in response to minor challenges. Combine that with external stressors and inconsistent sleep, and NPY becomes a daily driver of cravings and weight gain.

High NPY levels are also linked to fat accumulation, particularly around the belly. This makes sense from an evolutionary perspective: stress means danger, so store energy for survival. But in modern life, where stress is chronic and famine is unlikely, this backfires.

So how do you reduce NPY and its effects?

- Lower overall stress. This is key. Deep breathing, meditation, journaling, and therapy all reduce NPY output.
- Eat consistently. Skipping meals or going too long without food triggers more NPY release.
- Increase protein and fiber. These help regulate appetite and blunt NPY's hunger signals.
- Prioritize restorative exercise. Overtraining can increase stress and NPY. Favor moderate movement and rest.
- Sleep. As with every hormone, poor sleep raises NPY. Protect bedtime like your well-being depends on it, because it does.

If cortisol is the accelerator for stress, NPY is the fuel system that keeps you revving, especially toward emotional eating. The solution isn't to white-knuckle through cravings. It's to understand their source and support your nervous system enough that it no longer thinks you're in survival mode.

7. Glucagon-Like Peptide-1 (GLP-1): The Blood Sugar & Appetite Regulator

Glucagon-Like Peptide-1, or GLP-1, is a hormone released in the gut after eating. It plays multiple roles in digestion and metabolism. GLP-1 helps slow down gastric emptying (so you feel full longer), enhances the body's insulin response (to manage blood sugar), and even communicates with the brain to reduce appetite. You've probably heard about it recently because it's the basis for many popular medications used to treat diabetes and obesity.

But GLP-1 isn't just for those with a medical diagnosis. It's a critical player in how your body regulates hunger, blood sugar, and fullness, all of which become more challenging during perimenopause.

As estrogen declines, insulin sensitivity drops, and blood sugar becomes harder to manage. That leads to bigger spikes and crashes, more cravings, and more fat storage. When GLP-1 is functioning properly, it helps smooth those blood sugar curves by stimulating insulin secretion at the right time and reducing post-meal spikes.

Additionally, GLP-1 suppresses appetite by acting on the hypothalamus, the part of your brain that controls hunger. This suppression is more effective after meals rich in protein, fiber, and healthy fat, which stimulate more GLP-1 release. Meals high in refined carbs and sugar, however, cause blood sugar spikes that bypass this regulatory loop, leaving you hungry again within a couple of hours.

GLP-1 also interacts with dopamine, contributing to that calm, satisfied feeling you get after a nourishing meal. This helps explain why certain foods leave you feeling satisfied and steady, while others leave you restless and reaching for a snack shortly after.

How to naturally support GLP-1:

- Eat more slowly, which improves hormone signaling between the gut and brain
- Choose meals rich in protein and fiber, especially at breakfast
- Avoid sugar-only meals (e.g., pastries, juice) that bypass GLP-1 and trigger rebound hunger
- Include healthy fats, which also boost GLP-1 and slow digestion
- Get daily movement, which improves GLP-1 response and overall metabolic function

GLP-1 is like your metabolic stabilizer. When it's supported, your hunger feels manageable, your blood sugar stays in range, and you naturally eat less without feeling deprived. In perimenopause, where cravings and crashes become more common, GLP-1 can be a powerful ally.

8. Cholecystokinin (CCK): The Fullness Trigger

Cholecystokinin, or CCK, is a hormone secreted by cells in the small intestine when you eat, especially when you eat protein and fat. CCK has two main jobs: first, it stimulates the gallbladder and pancreas to release bile and digestive enzymes; second, and more importantly for perimenopause, it tells your brain that you're full.

CCK is one of the earliest hormones to respond during a meal. It starts signaling satiety within 15–20 minutes of eating, long before your stomach is actually full. When working properly, CCK helps prevent overeating and gives your brain a head start in turning off the hunger signal. But when your hormones are out of balance, CCK may become less efficient.

In perimenopause, this system can become desensitized. Shifts in estrogen, gut health changes, and altered bile production may reduce your ability to produce or respond to CCK. That means you may not register fullness until much later, or you may not feel satisfied at all. This delay is one reason why many women report overeating more often or needing larger portions to feel full.

Another issue is how quickly we eat. CCK is time-sensitive. If you inhale your meal in 5–10 minutes, CCK doesn't have time to fully activate. Slowing down allows it to do its job. It's also more effective when you chew thoroughly and include fats and protein in your meal.

CCK also plays a small role in managing cravings. Because it helps regulate dopamine (your brain's reward chemical), it can curb the drive to snack for emotional comfort, especially late at night when ghrelin tends to rise.

How to support CCK during perimenopause:

- Eat slowly, aiming for meals that last at least 20 minutes
- Include healthy fats (like avocado, nuts, or olive oil) and protein with each meal
- Chew your food thoroughly to stimulate the CCK response
- Avoid highly processed foods, which confuse or bypass your natural satiety signals
- Improve digestion by supporting gut health with fiber, probiotics, and gentle movement after meals

CCK is a quiet but powerful hormone. When functioning well, it allows you to stop eating comfortably, without needing willpower. When out of balance, it makes portion control feel impossible. In midlife, small shifts in how you eat can make CCK work for you again.

9. Pancreatic Peptide YY (PYY): The Long-Lasting Satiety Hormone

PYY, or Peptide YY, is released in the lower intestine after eating, particularly in response to protein and fat. Think of PYY as the hormone that sustains fullness. It doesn't kick in as fast as CCK, but it helps keep you satisfied long after a meal ends.

In perimenopause, many women find that meals don't "hold them" the way they used to. You may eat what feels like a solid breakfast, only to find yourself hungry again an hour later. That's where PYY may be underperforming.

Like GLP-1 and CCK, PYY helps reduce appetite, slows digestion, and contributes to overall food satisfaction. It works by acting on the hypothalamus to reduce hunger signals and by slowing gastric emptying, so your stomach stays full longer.

However, hormonal fluctuations, poor sleep, stress, and blood sugar instability can interfere with PYY release. If your meals are low in protein or too reliant on simple carbs, your PYY levels may not rise high enough to suppress appetite effectively. In addition, gut health plays a role. Since PYY is released from the intestine, imbalances in your gut microbiome can reduce its effectiveness.

PYY is also sensitive to meal size and spacing. Eating too frequently (grazing all day) or skipping meals completely can flatten your PYY rhythm. This is why structured meals with adequate portions, not just snacking, tend to improve appetite control over time.

Ways to support healthy PYY levels:

- Eat larger, balanced meals that include enough protein and healthy fat
- Avoid grazing, which reduces PYY's natural rhythm
- Incorporate soluble fiber, such as oats, apples, or flaxseed, to support digestion and satiety
- Focus on gut health with fermented foods, hydration, and prebiotic-rich vegetables
- Get regular movement, which improves gut function and hormone signaling

When PYY is working well, your body stays nourished and full between meals. You're less likely to snack unnecessarily or feel energy crashes. In a time when hunger can feel unpredictable and intense, PYY helps bring back consistency and calm.

2. What Mood Swings Really Mean

Let's be honest, midlife moods can be confusing. One moment you feel steady and grounded, and the next, something tiny sets you off. You snap at your partner. You burst into tears during a commercial. You feel anxious for no clear reason.

And then comes the guilt. Why am I so emotional? Why can't I just handle things like I used to?

Here's the truth: it's not you. It's your hormones. And more specifically, it's estrogen and its deep connection to your brain chemistry.

Estrogen plays a key role in regulating serotonin and dopamine, your body's natural mood boosters. These are the chemicals that help you feel balanced, upbeat, and capable. When estrogen levels fluctuate, as they do constantly during perimenopause, so does your access to those feel-good neurotransmitters. That's why your emotional floor can drop out even when nothing obvious has gone wrong.

This hormonal rollercoaster doesn't just impact your mood. It also affects how you respond to stress, how well you sleep, and how quickly you bounce back from frustration. And if you've been experiencing persistent irritability, sadness, or tension that feels "off," it's worth paying attention. These are not signs of weakness. They're hormonal clues.

Now for the empowering part: food can help. Certain nutrients support your mood-regulating systems, which means the meals you eat can either make the ride smoother or bumpier.

Some of the most effective mood-friendly foods include:

- Leafy greens like spinach and Swiss chard: rich in magnesium and folate
- Fatty fish like salmon and sardines: loaded with omega-3s
- Nuts and seeds, especially flax and pumpkin seeds: help balance hormones and ease anxiety
- Eggs: high in choline, which supports brain function
- Berries and citrus fruits: filled with vitamin C and antioxidants
- Dark chocolate (in moderation): a satisfying magnesium source with mood-enhancing compounds

And don't forget the importance of blood sugar balance. Sharp crashes caused by skipping meals or eating too many refined carbs can make your emotions spike and drop, just like your energy. When your brain doesn't get steady fuel, it doesn't function at its best.

This is not about "clean eating" or perfection. It's about giving your brain and body what they need to do their job, especially when your hormones are shaking things up.

3. Lifting the Fog: Nutrition for Mental Clarity

If you've ever walked into a room and completely forgotten why, or reread the same paragraph three times without absorbing it, welcome to the fog. Brain fog is one of the most frustrating symptoms of midlife, and you're definitely not imagining it.

This isn't a memory disorder. It's more like someone threw a light blanket over your thoughts. You're still sharp underneath, but things take more effort. You lose your train of thought. You misplace words. And sometimes you just feel... slow.

So what's going on?

Like mood, brain fog is directly connected to hormone levels. Estrogen supports the brain's blood flow and helps with communication between neurons. When estrogen fluctuates or drops, so does your brain's efficiency. Less blood flow means less oxygen and glucose to your brain cells, and that means slower recall, less focus, and more distraction.

But again, you're not stuck with this. What you eat has a massive impact on how clearly you think.

Here are some brain-boosting nutrients and where to find them:

- Choline, found in eggs, supports memory and mental clarity
- Omega-3s, found in fish, walnuts, and flaxseed, nourish your brain tissue
- Antioxidants, found in blueberries, green tea, and dark leafy greens, protect your brain from inflammation
- Complex carbs like quinoa, sweet potatoes, and oats give your brain steady fuel
- B vitamins, found in legumes, meat, and whole grains, support energy and concentration

And while we're talking clarity, let's not overlook the most basic factor: hydration. Even slight dehydration can affect your ability to think and focus. Many women mistake dehydration symptoms for fatigue, irritability, or forgetfulness.

A few smart hydration tips:

- Start your day with a glass of water before coffee
- Carry a water bottle and flavor it with lemon or cucumber if plain water bores you
- Eat water-rich foods like cucumbers, oranges, and melons

Just these small shifts, like hydration, whole foods, and fewer processed carbs, can help clear the fog that's been hanging over your brain for months.

4. Sleep, Cravings, and the Hormonal Domino

One of the sneakiest things about hormone shifts is how they mess with sleep. Maybe you fall asleep just fine, but wake up at 2 or 3 a.m. with your heart racing. Or maybe you sleep for eight hours but still feel groggy in the morning. Either way, poor sleep makes everything harder—your mood, your energy, your focus, and definitely your cravings.

Lack of sleep triggers your cortisol and increases your ghrelin, the hormone that makes you hungry. At the same time, it suppresses leptin, the one that tells you you're full. The result? You crave sugar, carbs, and comfort foods, not because you're weak, but because your hormones are pushing you toward quick energy.

Now, let's not pretend life allows for perfect sleep all the time. But what you can do is reduce the damage.

Some strategies include:

- Stop eating about 2–3 hours before bed so your digestion doesn't interfere with melatonin

- Avoid caffeine after 2 p.m., even if you think it doesn't affect you, it still raises cortisol
- Support your sleep with magnesium, found in nuts, seeds, leafy greens, and even a warm Epsom salt bath
- Try herbal teas like chamomile or lemon balm in the evening

Also, remember that eating regular meals with enough protein and healthy fats throughout the day helps stabilize blood sugar and reduces those 3 a.m. wake-ups caused by a dip in glucose.

Lastly, bring in some calming rituals. Journaling, stretching, and shutting off screens an hour before bed may sound small, but over time, they retrain your nervous system to settle down.

5. From Quick Fixes to Long-Term Wellness

If you've ever tried a 30-day detox, cut out entire food groups, or jumped into a strict eating plan with high hopes, you already know this story. It starts with motivation, maybe even results in the first week or two. But then comes the crash. The cravings return. Your energy drops. You feel deprived. And eventually, it all slips away.

The problem isn't your willpower. It's the wrong approach for your biology.

Midlife requires a different kind of wellness plan. One that respects your hormones, supports your stress levels, and works with your metabolism rather than trying to dominate it.

The truth is, most traditional diet programs were never built for women over 40. They weren't designed with fluctuating estrogen, increased cortisol sensitivity, or insulin resistance in mind. They were built around calorie math, not chemistry.

So what happens when you go low-fat, high-cardio, and calorie-obsessed during this chapter of life? You often end up hungrier, moodier, more bloated, and more discouraged. You may lose a little weight, but gain it back quickly. Your sleep gets worse. Your energy nosedives.

What works better?

- Eating more real food, not less
- Focusing on nutrients instead of numbers
- Prioritizing anti-inflammatory meals that calm the body
- Learning how to eat for hormonal rhythm, not just hunger

This is where food stops being about control and starts being about partnership. You're not fighting your body. You're finally feeding it what it actually needs to function.

6. Inflammation: The Hidden Hormonal Enemy

Let's take a closer look at one of the biggest disruptors of midlife wellness: inflammation.

Inflammation isn't just about sore joints or bloating. It's a full-body condition that can silently disrupt your digestion, mood, weight, skin, and even your brain. And during perimenopause and menopause, your risk of chronic low-grade inflammation rises dramatically.

Why?

Because declining estrogen means your natural anti-inflammatory protection weakens. Estrogen used to help regulate your immune response and protect your tissues from overreacting. Without it, your body becomes more sensitive to triggers, like sugar, poor sleep, stress, processed foods, and even excessive exercise.

The result? Your immune system stays "on," and you start feeling symptoms like:

- Constant fatigue
- Brain fog
- Digestive discomfort
- Puffy skin or swollen hands
- Sudden food sensitivities
- Stubborn belly weight that doesn't respond to diet or exercise

The solution isn't a cleanse or a crash. It's a consistent anti-inflammatory lifestyle, starting with food.

Key anti-inflammatory foods to prioritize:

- Leafy greens like kale, spinach, and arugula
- Colorful veggies like bell peppers, carrots, and beets
- Fatty fish like salmon and mackerel
- Berries, especially blueberries and raspberries
- Turmeric, ginger, and cinnamon for spice-based support
- Nuts and seeds, especially walnuts and flaxseed
- Olive oil as a primary fat

And just as important as what you add in is what you reduce:

- Refined sugar and sugary drinks
- Ultra-processed snacks
- Hydrogenated oils and trans fats
- Alcohol (especially in excess)
- Excess caffeine or energy drinks

This isn't about banning foods forever. It's about finding your body's calm. When inflammation lowers, everything else becomes easier—sleep, focus, weight loss, and even mood.

7. Support Beyond the Plate

Now that you understand how food connects to your hormones and inflammation, it's time to zoom out a bit. Because your lifestyle habits are just as important as your meals.

Your stress levels, daily movement, and even who you spend time with can either help regulate your hormones or throw them further off course.

Here's what to focus on:

1. Stress Management

Chronic stress raises cortisol, which disrupts nearly every other hormone. And let's face it, midlife is often full of responsibilities, like family, work, aging parents, shifting identities.

You don't need to eliminate stress. You need outlets. Gentle exercise, deep breathing, journaling, laughter, sunlight, time in nature, and genuine connection are not luxuries. They're hormone therapy in disguise.

2. Movement That Heals

Gone are the days when long, punishing cardio sessions were the goal. Midlife bodies thrive on a combination of strength training, walking, stretching, and restorative movement.

Why strength training? Because it helps you preserve lean muscle, boosts metabolism, supports bone density, and regulates blood sugar, all critical after 40.

Why walking? Because it gently lowers cortisol and clears mental clutter.

Why yoga or stretching? Because your nervous system needs calm just as much as it needs strength.

3. Boundaries and Rest

This is a season to learn how to say no. To recognize that pushing through isn't always the strong choice. Sometimes rest is the most radical decision you can make.

Give yourself space. That could mean time away from screens, taking a nap, or protecting your bedtime the way you'd protect a child's.

Remember, hormones heal best in a calm, well-fed, well-rested body. And you deserve that kind of care.

CHAPTER 3: PREPARE TO CHANGE YOUR LIFE

Before you change your body, you have to prepare your mind. That may sound cliché, but it's one of the most powerful truths I've seen play out again and again in women who succeed with the Galveston Diet. This chapter isn't about the food yet. It's not about the fasting windows, the meal prep, or even the weight loss. It's about getting your head in the right place to make this journey not just effective, but sustainable and empowering.

Here's the thing: most of us want transformation to happen overnight. We want the plan, the grocery list, and the fast results. That urgency is real, especially when you're exhausted, bloated, foggy, or fed up with the scale. But this process only works when it starts with clarity, not chaos. That's why this chapter exists, to slow things down so you can speed up later, more confidently and with much less frustration.

You don't need to be perfect. You don't need to feel 100 percent ready. And you definitely don't need to have it all figured out. But what you do need is a shift in mindset, a decision to approach this phase with curiosity instead of judgment. You are entering a new stage of life that requires a new way of eating, moving, and thinking.

There may be fear. There may be self-doubt. You may worry that this will be like every other time you tried and stopped. That's okay. Instead of trying to silence those feelings, I want you to expect them and bring them with you. The goal here isn't to pretend you don't have doubts. It's to keep going even with them.

So let's take a pause before we press forward. Before we start planning your meals or outlining your fasts, I want you to get grounded. This is where we start. Not with willpower, but with awareness.

1. Get Grounded: Know Where You're Starting

If you're serious about changing your health, you need a clear snapshot of where you're starting from. Not to judge yourself, but to give yourself a baseline. Otherwise, how will you know what's working?

Women often get hung up on the number on the scale, but I'm here to tell you, the scale is just one data point. Your body is going to shift in many ways on this plan, and some of the most exciting changes might not show up in pounds. That's why this step is so important: we're going to measure your progress from multiple angles.

Weight: Break Up with the Scale (But Take the Number)

Yes, I want you to weigh yourself. But just once, for now. Record it in a notebook along with the date. That's it. Then I want you to mentally "break up" with the scale. It's not your enemy, but it's not your coach either. It can't measure your muscle gain, your energy levels, your mental clarity, or your confidence. And it certainly can't measure your health.

As your hormones rebalance and your metabolism shifts, you may lose inches even if the number on the scale doesn't move. That's because you're likely gaining lean muscle while losing fat. Muscle weighs more than fat, but it takes up less space. So don't let the scale tell the whole story. Let it be a reference point, not a ruling.

Circumference Measurements

Next, take out a soft tape measure (cloth or flexible plastic) and measure:

- Waist: Find the narrowest part of your torso, usually just above the navel. Exhale gently and measure without sucking in.
- Hips: Measure the widest part of your hips and buttocks.
- Inner Thighs: Wrap the tape around the midpoint of one thigh.

Tip: Take measurements in front of a mirror to make sure the tape is level. And do it first thing in the morning, before eating or drinking anything, for consistency.

Waist-to-Hip Ratio (WHR): The True Health Indicator

The waist-to-hip ratio is one of the strongest indicators of visceral fat, the fat that sits around your internal organs and increases your risk for heart disease, diabetes, and cancer. Here's how to calculate it:

WHR = Waist circumference ÷ Hip circumference

Write that number down in your notebook. Then compare it to this chart:

WHR	Health Risk
0.80 or lower	Low
0.81–0.85	Moderate
0.86 or higher	High

Why does this matter? Because even if your weight doesn't change drastically, your WHR might drop significantly, showing you're losing dangerous fat and building better health.

Progress Photos: Not for Vanity, but for Victory

This step might feel awkward, but do it anyway: take a photo of yourself from the front, side, and back. Wear fitted clothing or underwear, stand in natural light, and try to keep the background and pose consistent. These photos are not about judging yourself, they're about having a visual timeline of change. You'll be amazed at the difference after four weeks, even if the scale hasn't budged.

You don't have to share these with anyone. Keep them in your notebook, journal, or private album. But take them. You'll be glad you did.

Start Tracking: Your Personal Health Ledger

Grab a small notebook or open a document on your phone or computer. This is now your health ledger, a place to track your weight, measurements, WHR, and photos. You'll revisit these metrics in four weeks. You don't have to track obsessively. You just need a baseline so that, when your energy improves, when your cravings calm, when your pants feel looser, you'll know exactly how far you've come.

2. Set Up Your Nutrition Toolkit

One of the biggest mindset shifts you'll make in this journey is understanding that tracking what you eat isn't about obsession, it's about awareness. When used properly, food tracking isn't about counting every crumb. It's about paying attention. And once you start paying attention, you take back your power.

Think of it like budgeting. You wouldn't try to improve your finances without first looking at your spending, right? The same logic applies to your nutrition. You don't have to track forever. But in the beginning, it's one of the most powerful tools you can use to understand your patterns and spot opportunities for improvement.

Best Apps for Tracking Macros and Nutrients

If you're new to food tracking, you'll want a simple, intuitive app that gives you insight into your macros (carbs, protein, fat) and micronutrients (vitamins, minerals, fiber). My top recommendation is Cronometer. It's one of the most accurate and comprehensive apps out there, with the ability to track net carbs (total carbs minus fiber) and customized macro goals.

Other solid options include:

- **Carb Manager:** especially useful if you're watching carbs
- **MyFitnessPal:** a longtime favorite with a large food database
- **Fitbit**: integrates with fitness tracking
- **Lose It!** and **MyNetDiary:** simple interfaces for beginners

Whichever you choose, look for the ability to track custom macros, view micronutrient breakdowns, and analyze net carbs, all central to the Galveston Diet.

Why Macros Matter More Than Calories

Here's the truth: not all calories are created equal. A 200-calorie protein-rich salad will impact your hormones, energy, and fullness very differently than 200 calories of cookies. That's why we focus on macronutrients, not calorie totals.

- Protein: crucial for muscle maintenance, satiety, and metabolism
- Healthy fats: essential for hormone production and brain health
- Fiber: improves digestion, balances blood sugar, and keeps you full

When your meals are rich in fiber, protein, and good fats, your body feels satisfied, and your cravings start to fade.

Original Idea #1: Weekly Food Reflection Prompts

In addition to logging your food, take 2 minutes each week to answer a simple prompt:

"How did the way I ate this week make me feel physically, mentally, and emotionally?"

This isn't about judging what you ate. It's about connecting the dots between food and how you function. Maybe you realize that skipping breakfast makes you foggy. Or that more vegetables leave you feeling clear-headed. These insights are the secret sauce to long-term change.

3. Build a Journaling Ritual

Nutrition tracking builds awareness of what goes into your body. But journaling builds awareness of what's happening inside your mind. Together, these tools create the foundation for behavior change.

Many women find that journaling helps them stay accountable, process emotions, and redirect self-sabotaging thoughts. You don't need to write a novel. Just a few minutes a day can shift your mindset dramatically.

Daily Journaling Prompts to Anchor Your Mindset

Here's a template to get started. Pick and choose the ones that resonate with you each day:

- Today I am grateful for:
- Two small self-care actions I'll take today:
- What I'm proud of from yesterday:
- My intention for today:
- One thing I'm letting go of today:
- My movement goal:
- My fasting window:
- Macros: carbs _____ fats _____ protein _____

Even if you write just one line per prompt, you'll be reinforcing a mindset of focus, grace, and progress, not perfection.

Original Idea #2: Monthly Progress Letters to Yourself

Every 30 days, set aside time to write a letter to yourself.

> What has changed in your *body*?
> What have you learned
> about your *eating patterns*?
> What *surprised* you, good or bad?
> What would you like to do
> *differently* next month?

These letters become a record of your evolution. And when you hit a tough week (and you will), you can look back at your own words and remember just how far you've come.

Freeform or Structured? Pick What Works for You

Some women thrive with structure. Others need a blank page. There's no wrong way to journal. Use a notebook, an app, a guided journal, or even the notes section on your phone. The important part is not how you do it, it's that you do it consistently.

Journaling is where you become your own best coach. It's where your "why" becomes clearer, your progress becomes visible, and your habits begin to root.

4. Smart Supplementation

Supplements can be incredibly helpful, but let's be clear: they're not a substitute for real food. Your plate should always be your first and best source of nutrition. Whole foods provide not only vitamins and minerals, but also enzymes, fiber, and phytochemicals that supplements simply can't replicate.

That said, during perimenopause and menopause, nutritional gaps are common. Many women struggle to meet daily needs for certain nutrients that support hormone balance, bone density, digestion, and brain function. The following three supplements are the ones I most often recommend to cover your bases and help smooth out the hormonal ride.

Fiber: Your Gut and Hormone Ally

Fiber does more than keep things moving. It helps balance blood sugar, supports gut health, and even binds to excess estrogen in the digestive tract, helping to eliminate it naturally.

There are two types:

- **Soluble fiber** (found in oats, chia seeds, psyllium): dissolves in water, slows digestion, and feeds healthy gut bacteria.
- **Insoluble fiber** (in vegetables, seeds, and whole grains): adds bulk and moves waste through your system.

You need 25–30 grams of fiber a day. Most women don't come close. That's why a supplement can help, especially if you're just starting to increase fiber intake.

Tips for choosing fiber supplements:

- Look for one with a blend of soluble and insoluble fiber.
- Avoid added sugars. Many flavored powders or gummies have as much sugar as candy.
- Start slow. Sudden increases can cause bloating or cramping.
- Take with a full glass of water and stay hydrated throughout the day.

Vitamin D: The Unsung Hormonal Hero

Vitamin D acts more like a hormone than a vitamin. It supports bone health, immune function, mood regulation, and yes, hormonal balance.

Your body makes vitamin D through sunlight exposure, but factors like age, skin tone, indoor lifestyles, sunscreen use, and geography can interfere. Many women are deficient and don't even know it.

Look for vitamin D3 (cholecalciferol)—the most bioavailable form. Doses between 1000–2000 IU per day are typical, but always check with your doctor and consider a blood test to determine your levels.

If you feel sluggish, down, or achy for no clear reason, low D might be part of the puzzle.

Omega-3s: Fuel for Brain, Hormones, and Inflammation

Omega-3 fatty acids are essential for managing inflammation, mood, cognitive function, and even hormone production. They're found in fatty fish (like salmon, sardines, mackerel), flaxseed, chia seeds, and walnuts, but it can be difficult to get enough through diet alone.

When choosing a supplement:

- Look for EPA and DHA (eicosapentaenoic and docosahexaenoic acid), the active forms
- Aim for at least 500 mg combined EPA + DHA per day
- If you're vegetarian or vegan, choose an algae-based omega-3 source
- Avoid supplements with added fillers or artificial flavors

Omega-3s support cell membrane integrity, brain health, and emotional regulation, which can be a game changer when your hormones feel like they're pulling you in five directions at once.

5. Hot Flash: Three Things You Should Do Right Now

If you're standing at the edge of a lifestyle change and wondering what's most important, start here. These three actions are the foundation for everything that follows. They're not about restriction or punishment. They're about supporting your body with what it actually needs.

1. Start Moving (Gently but Consistently)

You don't need a perfect gym routine or a personal trainer to start reaping the benefits of movement. Aim for 3–5 sessions per week, combining:

- Resistance training (to protect muscle and bone)
- Cardio (to support heart health and boost endorphins)
- Walking or stretching (to calm your nervous system)

Movement improves insulin sensitivity, mood, digestion, and sleep. It's not a punishment. It's medicine.

2. Upgrade Your Nutrition (One Choice at a Time)

Begin replacing processed foods with whole, nutrient-rich options. Focus on protein, fiber, and healthy fats. Drink more water. Cut back on sugar and alcohol where possible. Don't aim for perfect. Aim for better than yesterday.

Every nourishing meal is a signal to your body that it's safe, supported, and ready to heal.

3. If You Smoke, Make a Plan to Quit

This may be the most powerful shift you can make. Smoking not only triggers early menopause but also lowers estrogen, increases hot flashes, and drastically raises your risk of osteoporosis, cancer, heart disease, and stroke.

If you're considering hormone replacement therapy, most doctors won't prescribe it to smokers, because nicotine interferes with hormone function.

If you're struggling, you're not alone. Seek out a cessation program or talk to your physician. Your future self will thank you.

6. Prime Your Environment for Success

You can have the best intentions in the world, but if your surroundings don't support your goals, it's going to feel like an uphill battle. Let's fix that.

Your Social Circle: Make the Shift Together

Your relationships impact your habits more than you think. We mirror the behaviors of the people around us, often without realizing it. That's why it's crucial to tell the people close to you what you're doing, and why it matters.

- Ask for their support
- Set clear boundaries (e.g., no food shaming or diet talk)
- Invite someone to do the Galveston Diet with you
- Join an online community or accountability group

You don't have to do this alone. In fact, you shouldn't.

Your Physical Space: Make It Work for You

Your home, especially your kitchen, can either reinforce your healthy choices or sabotage them. Let's get it working in your favor.

Clean Out the Clutter

- Remove processed snacks, sugary temptations, and anything that doesn't align with your goals
- Give away or donate shelf-stable foods that are no longer part of your plan
- If others in your household eat differently, designate a separate shelf or drawer for their items

Stock the Essentials

Make sure your kitchen includes:

- Plenty of vegetables, fruits, lean protein, and healthy fats
- Quick, on-plan snacks like hard-boiled eggs, nuts, hummus, and chopped veggies
- Glass containers or meal prep kits for easy access and leftovers

Meal Prep: Start Small

You don't need to prep every bite of food for the week. But washing your produce, batch-cooking a protein, or making a soup or stew on Sunday can change the game.

And remember: prepping doesn't have to be perfect. It just has to reduce friction. The easier it is to make the right choice, the more often you will.

Creating a supportive environment means that healthy choices become easier, not harder.

7. Rehearse Your Plan Mentally

There's a reason elite athletes visualize their races, their shots, or their game days before they ever step into the arena. The mind is a powerful training ground. By mentally rehearsing your plan before you begin, you reduce uncertainty, lower resistance, and prepare yourself to succeed, even when things don't go perfectly.

This isn't wishful thinking. It's mental priming, and it works.

Before you officially start the Galveston Diet, take 5–10 minutes to walk yourself through your ideal day on the program. Close your eyes. Take a few slow breaths. Then imagine the following:

- **What time do you wake up?** Picture yourself getting up feeling clear and committed. You drink water. Maybe you do a short stretch or take a quiet moment before your day begins.

- **When does your fasting window begin and end?** Visualize how you feel during your fasting hours—occupied, energized, not deprived. Then imagine breaking your fast with a balanced, nourishing meal.

- ***What do you do when temptation shows up?*** Maybe it's cookies in the break room. Maybe it's a stressful moment when you want to snack. Picture yourself pausing, taking a breath, and choosing differently.

- **How do you respond when you feel tired or unmotivated?** Visualize your future self encouraging you to take just one small step. Prep a meal, journal, go for a walk.

- **How do you wind down at night?** Picture yourself finishing the day proud of your effort, no matter how small. You prepare for sleep feeling satisfied, not stressed.

The more often you rehearse this sequence, the more familiar it becomes. When the moment comes, you won't feel as unsure. You'll feel like you've already lived it.

Mental rehearsal is not about being perfect. It's about building confidence and trust in your ability to follow through, even on imperfect days.

By pausing here, by taking the time to measure, reflect, track, journal, and rehearse, you're not delaying your results. You're accelerating your success. In the same way a solid warm-up primes your body for movement, this preparation primes your mind for transformation.

Think of this chapter as your launchpad. Every note in your journal, every meal you track, every morning you rehearse your plan, it all stacks up. Little by little, you're stepping into the healthiest, most empowered version of yourself.

Take your time now so the rest of the journey can move with clarity and ease.

When you're ready, set your official start date. Circle it in your calendar. Write it in your journal. But don't skip this stage. Let it serve you fully.

Now let's move forward. The tools are here. The support is waiting.

And your next chapter is ready to begin.

PART TWO: THE RESET METHOD

CHAPTER 4: TIMED EATING FOR TIMELESS BENEFITS

In your 20s and 30s, skipping a meal or grabbing whatever was in the pantry may not have had lasting consequences. But now? Your body notices everything. The bloating. The cravings. The sluggish afternoons. Welcome to midlife metabolism, where when you eat becomes just as important as what you eat.

This is where timed eating, also called intermittent fasting, comes into play. And before you worry, no, this isn't about starving yourself or white-knuckling through hunger. It's about restoring a natural rhythm to your eating habits. A rhythm that honors your hormonal changes, supports fat loss, and helps reset your metabolism without overcomplication.

Let's begin with what it is, and what it's not.

1. What Is Timed Eating?

Timed eating is the practice of limiting your eating to a specific window of time each day and fasting (not eating) the rest of the time. For example, you might eat only between 12 p.m. and 8 p.m., and fast from 8 p.m. until noon the next day. That's a 16:8 approach, 16 hours of fasting, 8 hours of eating.

This isn't about drastically cutting calories. It's about giving your digestive and hormonal systems a consistent break, allowing them to function better with less metabolic stress.

There are different ways to structure timed eating:

- 12:12 - 12 hours of eating, 12 of fasting (a great place to start)
- 14:10 - 14 hours fasting, 10 hours eating (ideal for early transition)
- 16:8 - 16 hours fasting, 8 hours eating (common in Galveston Diet)
- 18:6 or 20:4 - Advanced strategies not ideal for early phases

The goal isn't to see how long you can go without food. The goal is to teach your body to burn fat for fuel, regulate hunger hormones, reduce inflammation, and stabilize blood sugar. Timed eating helps retrain your metabolism to be more flexible, switching between using glucose and fat as needed.

Let's be honest, midlife is when metabolism tends to slow down and fat loss becomes tougher. Timed eating offers a powerful reset, especially for women dealing with estrogen fluctuations, insulin resistance, and cortisol imbalance.

What It Isn't

Let's clear up a few common myths:

- It's not starvation. You're still eating satisfying meals during your eating window.
- It's not about skipping nutrition. In fact, the quality of your food still matters a lot.

- It's not a quick fix. It's a long-term metabolic strategy designed to work with your hormones, not against them.
- It's not for everyone in the same way. Some women thrive on 16:8, others feel better with a gentler 14:10. There's room for customization here.

Most importantly, timed eating fits within the framework of real life. You don't have to count points or log every bite. You simply eat during a window, and let your body handle the rest.

2. How Timed Eating Supports Hormone Balance

Now let's talk hormones, because everything we do in midlife nutrition comes back to the hormonal landscape. Timed eating actively impacts insulin, cortisol, ghrelin, leptin, and growth hormone, the very messengers that shape how you store fat, how often you're hungry, and how much energy you have.

Insulin: Your Fat Storage Regulator

One of the most powerful effects of timed eating is its impact on insulin sensitivity. In perimenopause and beyond, many women become more insulin-resistant, which means their cells no longer respond to insulin efficiently. This leads to higher blood sugar, more fat storage, especially around the belly, and stronger cravings for carbs.

By giving your body longer breaks between meals, insulin levels have time to drop and reset. This enhances your sensitivity and encourages your body to burn stored fat for energy instead of just glucose from food.

Put simply: when insulin is high, you're in storage mode. When insulin drops, you enter burn mode. Timed eating helps you spend more time in burn mode.

Cortisol: Calm the Chaos

Cortisol is your stress hormone, and it tends to run high when you're underslept, overwhelmed, or inflamed. Elevated cortisol contributes to fat storage, especially around the waist, and can keep your body in a chronic fight-or-flight state that suppresses digestion and disrupts sleep.

Timed eating, especially when paired with stable, anti-inflammatory meals, helps lower cortisol by reducing insulin spikes, improving sleep quality, and minimizing digestive stress. When your body isn't constantly processing food, it can prioritize rest, repair, and hormone regulation.

Leptin and Ghrelin: Hunger and Fullness Reset

Leptin is your satiety hormone. Ghrelin is your hunger hormone. Both often go haywire in midlife, especially when sleep is poor and meals are erratic. You feel hungry when you don't need food, and unsatisfied even when you've just eaten.

Timed eating helps restore the natural rhythm of these hormones. With consistent fasting and eating windows, ghrelin levels normalize, and you stop feeling like you need to graze all day. Leptin signals become stronger, helping you feel full and satisfied.

You're not fighting cravings anymore, you're retraining them.

Human Growth Hormone (HGH): Your Cellular Rejuvenator

During fasting, your body increases production of growth hormone, a key player in fat metabolism, muscle maintenance, and cellular repair. It's like pressing the reset button on your tissues.

In younger years, HGH is abundant. But as we age, it declines, unless you take specific actions to stimulate it, like strength training, quality sleep, and yes, fasting.

Timed eating gives your body space to do "behind-the-scenes" maintenance: detoxing cells, repairing damage, and cleaning up inflammation. All of this improves hormonal communication and reduces aging-related decline.

3. Benefits for Midlife Metabolism and Fat Loss

By the time you reach your 40s and 50s, it can feel like your metabolism has turned against you. Suddenly, the things that used to work, like cutting back on calories, hitting the gym hard, skipping dessert, don't seem to make a difference. Fat clings more stubbornly, especially around the belly. Your energy dips more often. And trying to "eat less and move more" just leaves you exhausted.

This isn't your fault. It's a hormonal shift. And timed eating is one of the most effective, science-backed strategies to realign your metabolism with your goals.

Why Fat Loss Is Harder After 40

A few things are happening all at once:

- Estrogen is declining, and that reduces your body's ability to burn fat efficiently
- Insulin resistance increases, making your body more likely to store fat instead of using it
- Cortisol rises, which triggers cravings and encourages belly fat
- Muscle mass drops, slowing your resting metabolic rate

That's a perfect storm for stubborn weight gain.

Timed eating helps by targeting the root of those changes. When you fast, insulin levels drop, and your body is encouraged to switch from storing to burning. You're no longer just burning calories from food, you're tapping into your own fat stores for energy.

This is called metabolic flexibility, your body's ability to move between fuel sources easily. In youth, this happens naturally. In midlife, it takes intentional effort. Timed eating gives your metabolism the nudge it needs.

You Burn More Fat, But Not Because You're Eating Less

One misconception about intermittent fasting is that it only works because you eat fewer calories. While it's true that many people naturally eat less when they reduce their eating window, the real magic is in hormonal timing.

With regular fasting, your body becomes more efficient at accessing stored energy. It learns to use fat as fuel, especially in the hours after your last meal. Studies show that fasting increases the activity of fat-burning enzymes and promotes lipolysis, the breakdown of fat cells.

And because growth hormone is elevated during fasting, you're also better able to maintain muscle mass, which is key for long-term metabolism and strength.

It Reduces Inflammation and Bloating

If you've felt puffy, bloated, or inflamed for no clear reason, fasting may help. Digesting food is energy-intensive and inflammatory for some people, especially when your meals are spaced out all day long.

Giving your gut a break for 12–16 hours allows it to rest, heal, and reduce systemic inflammation. This often leads to better digestion, clearer skin, and less fluid retention.

You Sleep Better, Too

When your last meal is earlier in the evening, your body can wind down without working to digest a late dinner or sugary snack. That means better melatonin production, fewer blood sugar crashes during the night, and improved sleep quality.

Sleep improves hormone regulation, which improves fasting success. It's a positive cycle.

A NOTE ON "FASTING CLEAN"

Can you have coffee during your fast?
What about tea, lemon water, or apple cider vinegar?
While everyone has their own version of what "breaks a fast," here's the general rule of thumb:
If it's under 50 calories, doesn't spike insulin, and doesn't contain protein or carbs, you're likely still in a fasted state.

So, during your fasting window, you can *usually enjoy*:

- Black coffee (no cream, no sugar)
- Herbal or green tea
- Water with lemon (but not lemon juice concentrate)
- Apple cider vinegar diluted in water
- Mineral water or seltzer

What to *avoid* during fasting:

- Bulletproof coffee or MCT oil (even though they're fat-based, they engage digestion)
- Bone broth (contains protein)
- Artificial sweeteners, which may confuse hunger and insulin signals

If your main goal is fat loss and insulin sensitivity, fasting clean keeps your body in its most metabolically active, fat-burning state. Once you break your fast, you want your first meal to be protein-rich and satisfying to reinforce the reset.

4. How to Ease Into Intermittent Fasting

One of the most important things I can tell you about starting timed eating is this: go slow. You are not behind. You're not in a race. And there's no bonus points for jumping straight into a 16:8 window if your body isn't ready.

Start with 12:12

A 12-hour fast and a 12-hour eating window is a gentle, sustainable way to begin. For example:

- **Finish dinner by 8 p.m.**
- **Eat breakfast at 8 a.m. the next morning**

That may not seem like much, but it resets your circadian rhythm, improves digestion, and begins building the habit of overnight repair.

Move to 14:10 When Comfortable

After a few days to a week on 12:12, try pushing your breakfast later. Stop eating at 8 p.m., and wait until 10 a.m. to have your first meal. That's 14 hours of fasting and a 10-hour eating window.

Most women feel great here, reporting improved focus, more energy, fewer cravings.

Advance to 16:8 If It Feels Right

If you feel steady at 14:10 and want to try 16:8, go for it. Stop eating at 8 p.m. and break your fast at noon. That gives you an 8-hour eating window (e.g., 12–8 p.m.) and a solid fasting period.

Again, you are not required to hit 16:8. If your schedule, stress levels, or sleep don't support it, 14:10 may be your sweet spot.

What to Eat When You Break Your Fast

Your first meal after fasting matters. Don't go straight to sugar, pastries, or simple carbs. These spike blood sugar and undo many of the benefits of your fasting period.

<u>Instead, break your fast with:</u>

- Protein: eggs, Greek yogurt, collagen smoothies, turkey, fish
- Healthy fats: avocado, olive oil, nuts
- Fiber-rich carbs: berries, leafy greens, chia, flaxseed

This combo calms hunger hormones, stabilizes energy, and helps you feel full for hours.

Listen to Your Body—but Don't Misinterpret It

The first few days may bring light hunger or early-morning cravings. That's normal. Your ghrelin rhythm is still adjusting. If you drink water, have a cup of tea, or distract yourself for 15–30 minutes, those sensations often pass.

But if you feel dizzy, irritable, or weak, then eat. This is about support, not suffering.

Over time, your body will shift into a new rhythm. Hunger won't feel urgent. Food will feel nourishing, not compulsive. And your metabolism will start responding like it wants to help you again.

5. Common Mistakes to Avoid

Intermittent fasting can be simple, intuitive, and incredibly effective, but only if it's approached with the right mindset. Too many women fall into the trap of doing it wrong, thinking they're helping their body when they're actually working against it.

If you want to get the most out of timed eating without the burnout, frustration, or hormonal backlash, here are some of the most common mistakes to avoid.

Mistake #1: Thinking Less Food = Better Results

This one's big. When you first start fasting, it's tempting to treat your eating window like a tiny space where you should squeeze in as little food as possible. But skipping meals or drastically under-eating can backfire hard.

If your body thinks it's being starved, it will slow your metabolism, increase cortisol, and cling to fat stores even more tightly. You may lose weight short term, but you'll feel awful, and you'll likely regain it.

What to do instead: Eat enough during your eating window. Focus on protein, fiber, and healthy fats. Satisfy your hunger so you're not white-knuckling your way through the fast.

Mistake #2: Ignoring Hydration

Your body does a lot of work during the fasting period. It cleans house, burns fat, balances hormones, and detoxifies. But it can't do those things efficiently if you're dehydrated.

Mild dehydration can lead to headaches, dizziness, irritability, and fatigue, all of which people often mistake as "fasting symptoms."

What to do instead: Aim to drink at least 60–80 ounces of water per day, and more if you're physically active. You can also sip on herbal tea, lemon water, or mineral water during your fast to stay refreshed.

Mistake #3: Breaking Your Fast With Sugar or Empty Carbs

One of the worst things you can do after fasting is break it with a high-sugar or processed-carb meal. Think: a muffin, a bagel, a sweetened coffee drink. Doing this causes a major insulin spike, which leads to a blood sugar crash, increased cravings, and stored fat.

What to do instead: Break your fast with balanced, nutrient-dense food, something with protein, healthy fat, and fiber. You want your body to feel stable, not shocked.

Examples:

- Eggs with avocado and sautéed spinach
- Greek yogurt with chia seeds and berries

- Salmon salad with olive oil dressing

Mistake #4: Skipping Sleep

This might seem unrelated, but sleep is one of the most important tools for fasting success. Poor sleep increases ghrelin (your hunger hormone), decreases leptin (your fullness hormone), and raises cortisol. That means more hunger, more cravings, and a higher likelihood of bingeing or breaking your fast early.

What to do instead: Prioritize sleep just like you prioritize your meals. Aim for 7–9 hours per night, and wind down without screens or late-night snacks. Fasting is easier and more effective when your nervous system is rested.

Mistake #5: Thinking Fasting Is All You Need

Intermittent fasting is powerful, but it's not a magic bullet. It won't undo a nutrient-poor diet, chronic stress, zero movement, or self-sabotaging patterns. Think of fasting as one pillar in a much bigger strategy.

What to do instead: Pair your fasting practice with clean eating, daily movement, emotional regulation, and supportive sleep. That's when the real transformation happens.

6. Sample Fasting Schedules for Midlife Women

One of the most empowering things about timed eating is that you can make it work for your lifestyle. There is no single "right" way to fast. The best approach is the one that fits your life, your energy levels, and your schedule.

Here are several realistic fasting schedules tailored to midlife women. Feel free to adapt them, blend them, or move between them based on your needs.

Option 1: 12:12 — The Gentle Beginning

- **Eating Window:** 8:00 a.m. – 8:00 p.m.
- **Fasting Window:** 8:00 p.m. – 8:00 a.m.

This schedule is perfect for women just starting out or those dealing with adrenal fatigue, chronic stress, or unstable blood sugar. It gives your digestive system rest without overwhelming your body.

Ideal for:

- Beginners
- Women with disrupted sleep
- High-stress seasons
- Anyone recovering from illness or burnout

Sample Day:

- 8:00 a.m.: Protein-rich breakfast (e.g., eggs + greens)

- 1:00 p.m.: Lunch (e.g., salmon salad)
- 6:30 p.m.: Dinner (e.g., chicken and roasted vegetables)
- 8:00 p.m.: Start fasting

Option 2: 14:10 — The Balanced Reset

- Eating Window: 10:00 a.m. – 8:00 p.m.
- Fasting Window: 8:00 p.m. – 10:00 a.m.

This is a great middle ground, long enough to boost fat burning and reduce insulin, but not so long that you feel deprived. Many women find 14:10 highly sustainable and energizing.

Ideal for:

- Most perimenopausal and menopausal women
- Moderate to high activity levels
- Anyone who's gone through 12:12 and wants more results

Sample Day:

- 10:00 a.m.: Break fast with Greek yogurt, berries, chia
- 2:00 p.m.: Lunch (e.g., chicken bowl with cauliflower rice)
- 7:30 p.m.: Dinner (e.g., grilled fish, leafy greens)
- 8:00 p.m.: Start fasting

Option 3: 16:8 — The Full Fasting Window

- Eating Window: 12:00 p.m. – 8:00 p.m.
- Fasting Window: 8:00 p.m. – 12:00 p.m.

This schedule provides a longer fasting window and is often used by experienced intermittent fasters. It stimulates more fat burning and more cellular repair through autophagy. You can move around the window, starting your Eating Window as early as 9 a.m. and ending it by 5 p.m.

Ideal for:

- Women who feel stable and energized with fasting
- Those looking to break through a fat-loss plateau
- Experienced Galveston Diet followers

Sample Day:

- 12:00 p.m.: Protein smoothie with greens and healthy fats
- 3:00 p.m.: Snack (e.g., boiled eggs, nuts, raw veggies)

- 7:30 p.m.: Dinner (e.g., grass-fed beef, sautéed kale)
- 8:00 p.m.: Start fasting

Note: If you're lifting weights or doing intense exercise, you may want to eat shortly after your workout, even if it breaks the fast.

Option 4: 5:2 Weekly Rhythm

- Structure: Eat normally five days per week, and reduce calories to 500–600 for two non-consecutive days

This model isn't time-restricted per day, but rather per week. It mimics traditional fasting without requiring daily changes.

Ideal for:

- Women with irregular schedules
- Those who travel frequently
- People who prefer flexibility over structure

Sample Week:

- Mon–Fri: Normal clean eating
- Tuesday and Saturday: 2 small meals totaling 500–600 calories

Note: This approach isn't as supportive of circadian rhythm repair as daily fasting but may be easier for women who want fewer constraints.

Option 5: Circadian Fasting

- Eating Window: Sunrise to sunset (usually 7:00 a.m. - 7:00 p.m.)
- Fasting Window: 7:00 p.m. - 7:00 a.m.

This rhythm aligns your meals with your natural light exposure, which supports hormone regulation, sleep, and digestion. It's an excellent option for women with high cortisol or insomnia.

Ideal for:

- Women with sleep issues
- Those who wake up hungry
- People trying to rebalance adrenal health

Sample Day:

- 7:00 a.m.: Oatmeal with chia, nuts, and protein
- 12:00 p.m.: Power lunch (e.g., turkey wrap with veggies)
- 6:30 p.m.: Light dinner (e.g., soup or salad with protein)

- 7:00 p.m.: Begin fast

Finding Your Fit

You don't have to commit to one schedule forever. Your fasting rhythm can shift based on your season of life, stress levels, energy needs, and even your cycle or travel.

Here's a suggestion:

- Start with 12:12 for 3–5 days
- Move to 14:10 for the next 1–2 weeks
- Try 16:8 if it feels energizing

Or settle into the version that best supports your life

Above all, listen to your body. You're not just resetting your eating—you're rebuilding trust with your metabolism.

7. How to Know It's Working

When you start a new routine like intermittent fasting, it's natural to look for quick signs that it's doing something. But unlike crash diets that promise overnight weight loss, timed eating works differently. It rewires your hormones, restores your metabolism, and teaches your body how to burn fat efficiently again. But it happens gradually, and some of the best indicators of success have nothing to do with the scale.

Here are the signs to look for that tell you timed eating is working, even if the number on the scale isn't moving (yet):

1. Reduced Cravings

One of the first and most powerful changes many women notice after a week or two of fasting is a significant drop in sugar and carb cravings. If you used to feel like you needed a snack every couple of hours or couldn't stop thinking about sweets in the afternoon, this alone can feel like a miracle.

Why it happens: Your insulin levels are dropping, your ghrelin rhythm is normalizing, and you're retraining your body to burn fat for fuel. That means fewer crashes, more steady energy, and fewer "give me chocolate or else" moments.

2. Mental Clarity and Focus

Brain fog is one of the most frustrating midlife symptoms. You walk into a room and forget why you're there. You can't remember words. You reread the same sentence five times.

One underappreciated benefit of fasting is its impact on mental sharpness. When you're in a fasted state, your body produces ketones, which your brain uses as a clean, efficient energy source. Many women report feeling more focused, alert, and creative after adopting a 14:10 or 16:8 window.

Look for moments in your day when you feel more "on." That's your brain responding to your body's metabolic reset.

3. Flatter Belly and Less Bloating

Even before fat loss begins, many women notice reduced bloating and inflammation in the first 7–10 days of fasting. This is due to lower insulin levels, better digestion, and fewer grazing opportunities that disrupt the gut.

If your clothes are fitting a bit better, your stomach feels less puffy, and you don't feel as sluggish after meals, that's a strong sign things are shifting in your favor.

4. More Stable Energy

No more rollercoaster energy. No more caffeine highs and carb crashes. Fasting helps you transition from being a sugar burner to a fat burner, which provides a steadier, longer-lasting energy source.

You may start to notice that:

- You feel more energized in the morning
- You don't "crash" midafternoon
- You can go longer between meals without feeling shaky or anxious

This is metabolic flexibility in action. Your body is finally burning the fuel it was designed to use.

5. You're Sleeping Better

Sleep and fasting are intimately linked. Once your eating window ends earlier in the evening, your body gets a clear circadian signal that it's time to wind down.

You may begin to fall asleep faster, stay asleep longer, and wake feeling more rested. Deep sleep is where hormone repair happens, so this is both a benefit of fasting and a fuel for further success.

6. You're Noticing Subtle Wins

Fasting isn't just about biology, it's also about rebuilding your relationship with hunger, food, and your own body.

Maybe you're starting to:

- Eat more mindfully
- Appreciate how good your body feels after a nourishing meal
- Set boundaries around food and work
- Feel more confident in your ability to follow through on your goals

These are wins. These are the moments that build real change. And they're just as valuable as any number on a scale.

8. When to Pause or Adjust Your Fast

One of the most empowering truths about timed eating is this: you are allowed to adapt it to your real life. This is not a rigid, one-size-fits-all rulebook. It's a tool, a flexible, powerful tool, and just like any tool, sometimes you need to adjust how you use it.

Here are situations where it's not only okay but wise to pause, modify, or completely change your fasting rhythm.

1. If You're Not Sleeping Well

Sleep is more foundational than fasting. If you're waking up at 3 a.m. every night, struggling to fall asleep, or feeling depleted, your body may need more nourishment earlier in the day or a gentler fasting window.

Try shifting from 16:8 to 14:10 or even back to 12:12. Prioritize sleep first. Once you're rested, fasting becomes more effective.

2. If You're Exercising Intensely

Strength training, running, or high-intensity interval training can require more frequent fueling, especially if you're lifting weights in the morning.

If your workouts leave you shaky or ravenous, consider eating a small, protein-rich meal before or after exercise, even if it slightly overlaps with your fast. Supporting your muscles is more important than sticking to a perfect clock.

3. If You're Under High Stress

Emotional, financial, or physical stress elevates cortisol, and layering fasting on top can sometimes make things worse. If fasting begins to feel like pressure, or if your hunger feels frantic or exhausting, take a break.

Stress management comes first. You can always return to a longer fast when life steadies out.

4. If You're in Your Luteal Phase (for Cycling Women)

For women who are still cycling, the luteal phase (after ovulation, before menstruation) is when progesterone rises and your metabolism speeds up slightly. Many women naturally feel hungrier during this time.

You don't have to fight it.

Instead, honor your body's signals. Ease into a 12:12 rhythm, increase protein and fat slightly, and prioritize calming rituals. After your period, you'll likely feel ready to resume a longer fast.

5. If You're Sick or Run Down

When you're recovering from illness, surgery, or a particularly exhausting week, fasting may need to take a back seat. Your immune system and adrenal glands require fuel and rest. The focus should be hydration, nutrient-dense meals, and sleep.

You're not "falling off." You're supporting healing, which is the point of this lifestyle in the first place.

How to Know When to Adjust

Ask yourself:

- Am I feeling strong and focused, or weak and foggy?
- Am I hungry in a calm way, or desperate and distracted?
- Is fasting helping my sleep and mood, or making it harder?
- Am I able to maintain this rhythm, or am I fighting it every day?

If your answers lean toward struggle, that's your cue to adjust.

Fasting works best when your body feels supported, not punished. It's not about pushing through hunger to prove something. It's about working with your body's needs, which change daily, weekly, seasonally.

You can shift your fasting rhythm as needed, and still make progress.

The Bigger Picture

Remember: the goal of fasting is not to eat as little as possible or follow a rigid clock. The goal is to build metabolic strength, reduce inflammation, balance hormones, and restore your energy.

That means eating nourishing food, listening to your body, and giving yourself grace to adjust as needed.

Some days, 16:8 will feel amazing. Other days, 12:12 will be plenty. The rhythm doesn't have to be perfect. It just has to be yours.

When in doubt, come back to your "why." You're doing this to feel better, think clearer, move easier, and live more fully. Fasting is just one path to get there, and now, you're equipped to walk it with clarity and strength.

CHAPTER 5: EAT TO COOL THE FIRE

Inflammation is a word we often associate with visible swelling, redness, or infection. You might picture a swollen ankle after a fall or a sore throat when you're coming down with something. That kind of inflammation is acute and helpful. It means your immune system is doing its job, rushing to the site of injury or infection to heal and protect you.

But there's another kind of inflammation. It's invisible, slow-burning, and far more dangerous. This is chronic inflammation, and for many women in midlife, it quietly becomes a major roadblock to health and vitality.

Chronic inflammation is like a constant low-level alarm going off inside your body. It may not cause sharp pain, but it wears down your systems over time. Instead of turning off once a threat has passed, your immune system stays activated. This leads to widespread effects that are often dismissed as "just getting older."

In reality, symptoms like belly fat that won't budge, joint pain, bloating, fatigue, hot flashes, and brain fog can all be linked to this internal fire. When inflammation is present, your body feels more tired, your metabolism becomes sluggish, and your hormones are harder to regulate.

During perimenopause and menopause, your body naturally becomes more vulnerable to this process. One key reason is the drop in estrogen, which has natural anti-inflammatory properties. Estrogen plays a role in keeping your blood vessels flexible, your immune system balanced, and your metabolism steady. As it declines, inflammation can increase without you even realizing it.

At the same time, other hormonal changes are happening. Insulin becomes less effective, making it harder for your body to regulate blood sugar. This leads to higher insulin levels, which in turn can feed inflammation. Cortisol, your primary stress hormone, also tends to rise in midlife. Chronic stress and poor sleep can keep cortisol elevated, which adds even more fuel to the inflammatory fire.

This isn't just uncomfortable. It's risky. Chronic inflammation is linked to serious long-term health issues, including heart disease, diabetes, autoimmune conditions, and even cancer. But for many women, it starts with everyday symptoms that feel frustrating and difficult to explain. You may feel tired even after a full night's sleep. You may notice weight gain, especially around your waist, that seems completely resistant to diet or exercise. You may feel more achy, more puffy, and more irritable, and you may not realize that inflammation is quietly behind the scenes.

The good news is that you can calm this fire. And one of the most powerful ways to do that is through your food. What you eat each day has the ability to either feed the flames of inflammation or help extinguish them. In this chapter, you'll learn how to use your plate as your healing tool.

Anti-inflammatory eating is not restrictive. It is nourishing, satisfying, and deeply aligned with what your body truly needs during this stage of life. And once you begin to eat this way, your symptoms won't just improve. You'll likely feel clearer, lighter, and more energized than you have in years.

1. How Food Fuels or Fights Inflammation

You've probably heard the word "inflammation" tossed around like it's the enemy of all things good. And in many ways, it is. Chronic inflammation acts like a low-level fire in your body, slowly damaging tissues, disrupting hormones, and exhausting your energy reserves. But what fuels this fire, and more importantly, what puts it out, can often be traced directly to what's on your plate.

Let's start with what fans the flames.

Pro-Inflammatory Foods: What to Minimize

Not all foods are created equal. Some sneak into your system like sugar-coated saboteurs, triggering internal alarms and keeping your immune system on edge. Refined carbohydrates, like white bread and pastries, break down quickly into sugar. That sugar spikes your insulin levels, which then signals your body to store fat and hold on to it. Over time, this leads to insulin resistance, weight gain, and—you guessed it—inflammation.

Then there's processed sugar in all its forms: syrups, sweetened drinks, and the "hidden sugar" in seemingly healthy foods like yogurts or salad dressings. Sugar disrupts your gut bacteria, promotes fat storage, and increases markers of inflammation in your blood. Even moderate consumption, if consistent, can send your body into a low-grade inflammatory state.

Processed oils are another hidden trigger. These include vegetable oils high in omega-6 fats, like soybean, corn, or sunflower oils, which can overpower the anti-inflammatory effects of omega-3s. When your omega-6 to omega-3 ratio is off balance, your body enters a pro-inflammatory state, making everything from joint pain to brain fog worse.

Let's not forget alcohol and chemical additives. Alcohol may seem harmless in small amounts, but regular consumption stresses your liver, disrupts hormonal balance, and weakens the gut lining. Artificial additives and preservatives can interfere with immune regulation and increase the toxic load your body must process.

Anti-Inflammatory Foods: Your Kitchen's Medicine Cabinet

Thankfully, food can also be your most powerful ally. Anti-inflammatory nutrition is all about choosing real, whole foods that nourish your body and keep inflammation at bay. It's less about restriction and more about direction, eating in a way that heals instead of harms.

Start with fiber-rich vegetables. Leafy greens like kale and spinach, cruciferous veggies like broccoli and cauliflower, and colorful options like carrots, beets, and peppers all help your gut produce short-chain fatty acids that reduce inflammation and support immune balance.

Healthy fats are another must. Think extra virgin olive oil, avocado, nuts, and seeds. These are rich in monounsaturated fats and antioxidants that protect cells from oxidative stress. Omega-3s found in fatty fish like salmon, sardines, and mackerel help reduce pro-inflammatory cytokines, making them one of the most potent inflammation fighters in your diet.

Lean proteins also matter. Choose wild-caught fish, organic poultry, pasture-raised eggs, and plant-based options like lentils or quinoa. These give your body the amino acids it needs for repair and balance without the inflammatory baggage that often comes with overly processed meats.

And then there are the flavor heroes: turmeric, ginger, garlic, cinnamon, and green tea. These natural anti-inflammatory agents have been used for centuries to reduce swelling, ease pain, and improve circulation. A little spice can go a long way toward healing.

The Gut–Inflammation Link: A Two-Way Street

Your gut is not just a digestion machine. It's home to trillions of microbes, many of which directly influence how your immune system reacts. An unbalanced gut microbiome can cause the gut lining to weaken, allowing unwanted particles to pass into the bloodstream and trigger inflammation. This condition,

> Every bite you take either feeds the fire of inflammation or helps put it out. Let your food be your hormone-supportive, energy-restoring medicine.

sometimes referred to as "leaky gut," has been linked to everything from fatigue and bloating to autoimmune disorders and hormonal chaos.

When you eat pro-inflammatory foods, you're not just irritating your system in the short term. You're changing your microbial environment, weakening your defenses, and inviting long-term damage. Anti-inflammatory foods, in contrast, help strengthen your gut lining, balance your microbiome, and reduce immune overactivation.

It's a daily choice. Every meal is an opportunity to reduce inflammation, calm your body, and reclaim your energy. There's no need to be perfect. Just intentional.

2. What Happens When You Start Eating to Heal

You don't have to wait months to feel the difference. When you begin eating with healing in mind, your body responds quickly and kindly. It's like shifting from chaos to calm. Healing foods don't just fill your stomach, they speak to your hormones, your cells, and your entire internal ecosystem.

Short-Term Benefits: The First Few Weeks

The early signs might surprise you. Within just a few days of ditching inflammatory foods and adding nutrient-rich meals, bloating begins to settle. Your digestion smooths out. You feel lighter, not just in weight, but in mood.

Your skin often reflects internal shifts. That redness, puffiness, or acne that once seemed stubborn may start to fade. You may wake up feeling clearer, not just in your face but also in your mind. Brain fog, once a constant cloud, begins to lift as inflammation cools and blood sugar stabilizes.

Many women also report a calmer emotional baseline. You may still feel stress, but it no longer hijacks your whole day. With fewer sugar crashes and better-regulated cortisol, your mood stays steadier and your responses more balanced. Emotional eating starts to lose its grip.

And energy? It starts to return. Not the jittery kind, but a grounded, sustained energy that gets you through the day without caffeine band-aids or late afternoon crashes.

Long-Term Impact: What Sticks and Builds

Beyond the immediate shifts, there's something even more powerful taking root. As your body adapts to consistent, healing nourishment, systems start to sync. Your hormones begin to regulate with less drama and more rhythm.

Fat loss becomes easier, not because you're starving or chasing numbers, but because your body is no longer inflamed or insulin resistant. When insulin sensitivity improves, your cells unlock fat more easily for energy use. The scale may move, but more importantly, your waistline reflects hormonal change.

Risk factors for chronic disease also begin to shrink. Anti-inflammatory foods help lower your chances of developing heart disease, type 2 diabetes, and certain cancers. When estrogen is detoxed efficiently and cortisol is stabilized, your entire endocrine system operates more smoothly.

Eating to heal is not just about avoiding illness. It's about thriving in your body. That sense of being "at odds" with yourself begins to fade. You start to feel like your body is finally on your side.

The Science of Why: Food and Hormone Chemistry

Behind all these visible changes is a quiet revolution happening in your bloodstream and your cells. Let's break it down.

When you eat low-quality food filled with sugar, additives, or inflammatory oils, your blood sugar spikes. That triggers insulin. Over time, too many spikes make your body numb to insulin's signal, leading to weight gain and constant fatigue. Eating fiber-rich, whole foods stabilizes blood sugar, lowers insulin demand, and reopens your body's natural fat-burning channels.

Cortisol, the stress hormone, also responds to food. Skipping meals or fueling on processed carbs can cause cortisol to surge, creating belly fat and sleep disturbances. Balanced meals with protein, healthy fats, and antioxidants help regulate this stress response. Your body begins to feel safe again, no longer in survival mode.

Estrogen detox is another hidden piece. Estrogen is meant to rise and fall in rhythm, but poor gut health and processed foods can slow down its clearance. This leads to estrogen dominance. Think heavy periods, stubborn fat, and mood swings. Healing foods support liver detox and feed the gut bacteria that help metabolize estrogen efficiently.

Your food choices are not just meals. They're messages. Each bite tells your hormones what kind of environment they're living in. The better the food, the clearer and kinder the signal.

3. Anti-Inflammatory Pantry Staples

Eating to heal becomes much easier when your kitchen is stocked with the right ingredients. A healing lifestyle doesn't start at your plate, it starts at the grocery store and lives in your pantry. Building an anti-inflammatory kitchen is like setting yourself up with a daily support system. You make healing convenient and inflammation inconvenient.

> Your pantry shapes your daily choices.
> Fill it with foods that help you heal,
> not ones that hold you back.

This section walks you through the must-have staples to keep on hand, so you're never more than a few steps away from a nourishing meal.

Anti-Inflammatory Fats: Your Hormone-Helping Heroes

Let's start with fats. Not all fats are created equal. Anti-inflammatory fats are rich in monounsaturated or omega-3 fatty acids, and they help build hormones, lower inflammation markers, and support brain and skin health.

Stock these regularly:

- **Avocados:** Rich in heart-healthy fats and potassium.
- **Extra virgin olive oil:** Best used cold or in low-heat cooking to preserve its antioxidant profile.
- **Nuts**: Especially almonds, walnuts, and Brazil nuts. A small handful gives you a nutrient boost with staying power.
- **Seeds**: Chia, flax, and hemp seeds are loaded with omega-3s and fiber.

Avoid seed oils like soybean, corn, and canola. These are high in omega-6 fats and can disrupt the delicate balance your body needs to keep inflammation in check.

Vegetables and Fruits: Fiber, Color, and Healing Power

No anti-inflammatory plan works without a wide variety of vegetables and fruits. These plant foods provide fiber, antioxidants, and polyphenols that cool inflammation from the inside out.

Focus on these categories:

- **Cruciferous veggies:** Broccoli, cauliflower, cabbage, and Brussels sprouts support estrogen detox and gut health.
- **Leafy greens:** Kale, spinach, arugula, and chard contain essential nutrients and help alkalize the body.
- **Deep-colored produce**: Berries, beets, red cabbage, and purple grapes offer powerful antioxidants that protect your cells from damage.
- **Alliums**: Garlic, onions, and leeks are anti-inflammatory and antibacterial.

Buy fresh, seasonal produce when possible, and supplement with frozen options to keep your freezer stocked and your meals colorful year-round.

Spices: The Secret Weapon in Your Cabinet

Healing doesn't have to be bland. Many spices have powerful anti-inflammatory properties and add depth to meals without relying on heavy sauces or sugars.

Always keep these close:

- Turmeric: Contains curcumin, which targets inflammation and joint pain. Pair it with black pepper for better absorption.
- Ginger: Soothes digestion and reduces oxidative stress.
- Cinnamon: Helps regulate blood sugar and adds warmth to both sweet and savory dishes.
- Garlic powder, cumin, paprika: Flavor enhancers with immune-boosting benefits.

Spices can turn a basic dish into something satisfying and medicinal. They're inexpensive, shelf-stable, and powerful.

Proteins: Clean and Balanced Sources

Your body relies on protein to rebuild tissue, regulate hormones, and keep your metabolism humming. But quality matters just as much as quantity.

Build your pantry and fridge with:

- Wild-caught fish: Especially salmon, sardines, and mackerel. Rich in anti-inflammatory omega-3s.
- Pasture-raised poultry: Lower in saturated fats and free of antibiotics and hormones.
- Legumes: Lentils, chickpeas, black beans. Great plant-based options that offer fiber, iron, and slow-digesting carbs.
- Organic eggs: High in choline and versatile across meals.

Look for organic, pasture-raised, and sustainable labels when possible. The cleaner the source, the less inflammatory stress your body has to deal with.

Grains and Legumes: Whole and Unprocessed

While grains can be controversial, the right ones can absolutely support an anti-inflammatory lifestyle, especially when paired with fiber and protein.

Best picks include:

- Quinoa: A complete protein and gluten-free grain that cooks quickly.
- Steel-cut oats: High in beta-glucans and help reduce cholesterol and regulate blood sugar.
- Lentils: A versatile pantry staple with both protein and fiber.
- Brown rice and wild rice: Better than white rice due to their intact bran layer and nutrients.

Avoid ultra-processed grain products like sugary cereals, white bread, and flavored instant oat packets. These can spike insulin and keep inflammation active.

Label-Reading Tips: Spotting Hidden Triggers

Even healthy-looking foods can hide inflammatory ingredients. Learning how to read labels gives you control and confidence.

Here's what to watch for:

- Added sugars: Look for words like glucose, corn syrup, dextrose, and maltodextrin.
- Inflammatory oils: Steer clear of anything listing soybean oil, corn oil, or hydrogenated fats.
- Artificial additives: Dyes, preservatives, and flavor enhancers can irritate your gut and overwork your immune system.
- "Natural flavors": This vague term can mask dozens of chemical compounds. It's not always harmful, but it's best to minimize.

A good rule of thumb: if you don't recognize it, your body probably doesn't either.

4. How to Build an Anti-Inflammatory Plate

It's one thing to know what foods are anti-inflammatory. It's another to put them together in a way that actually fuels your body and fits your life. This is where the Galveston Diet plate method comes in. It's simple, flexible, and powerful enough to support hormone health, metabolism, and long-term fat loss.

Eating anti-inflammatory meals isn't about chasing perfection. It's about building balance. When your plate supports healing and hormone regulation, everything else gets easier—your energy, your digestion, your mood, and your cravings.

The Galveston Diet Plate Method

Picture your plate as a circle divided into thoughtful sections. This visual method ensures you're getting the right macronutrient balance while focusing on foods that cool inflammation rather than fuel it.

Here's the basic structure:

- Half your plate should be non-starchy vegetables. Think leafy greens, cauliflower, zucchini, bell peppers, asparagus, and mushrooms. These provide fiber, antioxidants, and volume without blood sugar spikes.
- One quarter should be lean protein. This could be wild-caught fish, pasture-raised chicken, organic tofu, or legumes. Protein supports muscle repair, keeps you full, and helps regulate cortisol.
- The final quarter is for healthy fats and slow-digesting carbs. Include foods like avocado, extra virgin olive oil, quinoa, lentils, or sweet potatoes. These round out the meal with sustained energy and hormone-building blocks.

This ratio helps calm your immune system, reduce cravings, and maintain blood sugar stability throughout the day. You won't feel the rollercoaster crash of refined carbs or the midday fog from a sugar-heavy lunch.

Balancing Macros with Inflammation in Mind

Macronutrients like protein, fat, and carbohydrates are more than calorie sources. They send messages to your hormones and influence how your body processes stress, stores fat, and heals from inflammation.

- Protein is critical after 40. It supports lean muscle, which helps burn fat and stabilize blood sugar. Aim for 20 to 30 grams per meal.
- Healthy fats are your anti-inflammatory allies. Monounsaturated fats from olive oil and avocado and omega-3s from fish and seeds help reduce joint pain, brain fog, and cortisol overload.
- Complex carbs provide fiber and fuel your microbiome. Choose options like lentils, steel-cut oats, or root vegetables instead of white rice or refined bread.

There is no need to fear carbs, but the type and timing matter. Pair carbs with protein or fat to slow digestion and reduce insulin spikes.

Sample Anti-Inflammatory Meals: Easy Ideas for Any Day

Need help visualizing your anti-inflammatory plate in action? Here are sample ideas that are balanced, satisfying, and simple to prepare:

- Breakfast:

Spinach and mushroom omelet cooked in olive oil, topped with avocado slices. Side of mixed berries and a sprinkle of ground flaxseed.

- Lunch:

Grilled salmon over arugula and quinoa, tossed with olive oil, lemon juice, pumpkin seeds, and roasted sweet potato cubes.

- Dinner:

Lentil and vegetable stew with garlic, turmeric, and cumin. Side of sautéed kale with toasted walnuts. Herbal tea with ginger.

- Snack:

Sliced apple with almond butter, or a boiled egg with cherry tomatoes and a handful of pistachios.

Keep meals colorful and season them well. The more vibrant your plate looks, the more antioxidants it likely contains. Spices like turmeric, ginger, and paprika not only flavor your meals but also enhance their healing properties.

How to Eat Out Without Sacrificing Your Goals

- Look for grilled, baked, or roasted proteins, not fried or breaded.
- Ask for dressing or sauces on the side. Many are loaded with sugar or seed oils.
- Swap out fries or white rice for extra veggies, side salads, or legumes.
- Watch your drinks. Alcohol, soda, and sweet teas can undo a balanced meal.

Life doesn't happen in a meal plan, so knowing how to eat out while staying aligned with your goals is essential. The key is to scan the menu for meals that resemble your anti-inflammatory plate.

You can also take control by eating a protein-rich snack before going out. This lowers the chance of impulsive choices made from hunger or low blood sugar.

If you indulge, do it with intention. One meal will not undo your progress. What matters is how you eat most of the time. When anti-inflammatory eating becomes your default, your body becomes resilient.

5. Common Roadblocks and How to Navigate Them

Starting a new way of eating can feel exciting at first. But real life always shows up—with cravings, chaos, and curveballs. Knowing what roadblocks to expect and how to move through them helps you stay on course without guilt or confusion. Here's how to tackle the most common challenges with confidence.

Sugar Withdrawal or Cravings

If your body has relied on sugar for years, the first few days of clean eating may bring headaches, mood dips, or irritability. This is your body recalibrating. You're not failing—you're detoxing.

Drink plenty of water. Eat more fiber and healthy fat. Snack on foods like avocado, hard-boiled eggs, or chia pudding to stay satisfied. Cravings tend to fade by day five, and when they do, your energy stabilizes like never before.

Family Members Not on Board

Maybe your partner still wants pizza or your kids roll their eyes at lentils. Don't let this stop your progress. Focus on meals you can all share with simple modifications. For example, make a taco night with both lettuce wraps and tortillas. Offer fruit instead of sugary desserts. Keep your staples visible and easy to grab.

You don't have to convince everyone to join. You just need to lead by example. Over time, they'll notice the changes in you—clearer skin, better mood, steady energy—and curiosity will follow.

Getting Overwhelmed in the Kitchen

You don't need to cook elaborate meals to eat anti-inflammatory. A meal can be as simple as roasted veggies, grilled protein, and olive oil drizzle. Batch-cook proteins and grains. Use spice blends to make even basic dishes flavorful.

Try preparing just two recipes for the week and rotating them. Keep frozen veggies and pre-cut ingredients on hand for backup. Start with what feels doable, then build from there.

Budget and Convenience Concerns

Yes, organic food and wild-caught fish can add up. But anti-inflammatory eating is scalable. Beans, lentils, frozen vegetables, and oats are affordable and nourishing. Shop in bulk when possible and prioritize ingredients that deliver multiple meals.

Avoid ultra-processed "health" foods with fancy labels. Real healing comes from simple ingredients. Make a grocery list before shopping, and don't underestimate the power of one-pot meals or slow cooker soups that stretch across several days.

Healing doesn't require perfection or expensive habits. It just requires consistency and kindness toward yourself.

6. So… What About Coffee, Wine, and Chocolate?

Let's be honest. Total deprivation rarely works for the long term. And if you're wondering whether there's room for your morning coffee, a glass of wine, or a bite of chocolate, there is. With a little mindfulness, you can enjoy these indulgences without sabotaging your healing.

Coffee

Good news. Coffee is not the enemy. In fact, it contains antioxidants and may even reduce inflammation in moderate amounts. But how you drink it matters. Skip the sugar-laden creamers and flavored syrups. Use a splash of unsweetened almond milk or a dash of cinnamon. If caffeine affects your sleep or cortisol levels, try limiting it to mornings or switching to half-caf.

Wine

Red wine, in moderation, can offer heart-healthy polyphenols like resveratrol. But alcohol still places a burden on your liver and can disrupt hormonal detox. Keep it to one glass a few times per week, preferably with food. If you're dealing with intense fatigue, hot flashes, or mood swings, consider taking a break and noticing how your body responds.

Chocolate

Dark chocolate with a high cacao content (70 percent or more) is rich in magnesium and antioxidants. One or two squares can satisfy a sweet craving without triggering blood sugar spikes. Look for options with minimal sugar and no dairy or soy fillers.

The key with all three is moderation and awareness. Know your triggers, check how your body reacts, and focus on quality over quantity.

Pleasure is not the enemy of healing. When you choose mindfully, these small indulgences can be part of your wellness—not a threat to it.

Healing doesn't happen in a single meal. It happens in the small choices you make day after day. The quiet decision to skip the sugary snack. The moment you reach for greens instead of chips. The mornings you hydrate before caffeinating. These are not grand gestures, but they add up. They whisper to your hormones that it's safe to reset, to balance, to heal.

Consistency matters far more than perfection. You don't need to be flawless. You just need to stay in motion. Your body is incredibly forgiving when you nourish it, even after years of neglect. Every anti-inflammatory meal is a message of support, a vote for your future self.

This is not a diet of deprivation. It's a daily act of partnership with your body. You are choosing foods that love you back. You're lowering inflammation, supporting your mood, and creating a foundation for better sleep, stable weight, and clearer thinking.

As you move into the next section, you'll discover that fat—once feared—is actually one of your most powerful allies. In the right forms, healthy fats can rebuild hormones, stabilize cravings, and fuel long-lasting energy. Get ready to welcome them back to your plate without guilt.

CHAPTER 6: FAT IS NOT THE ENEMY

For decades, we were told to fear fat. Skim milk was good. Bacon was bad. Salad dressing came with a warning label. The shelves were lined with low-fat, fat-free, and "light" products that promised health and weight loss. But here's the uncomfortable truth: that era didn't make us healthier. It made us tired, inflamed, and confused. For many women over 40, it also made midlife weight gain feel like a personal failure.

The real problem wasn't the fat. It was the story we were told about it.

Your body after 40 is not the same body you had in your twenties. Your hormones are shifting. Estrogen is declining. Cortisol is rising. Insulin sensitivity is changing. And the nutritional needs of your body are evolving too. What worked before may not only stop working, it may actually make things worse. That's why unlearning old diet rules becomes just as important as learning new ones.

This chapter is about giving fat its rightful place back at the table. But it's also about fiber and protein—two other key players that often get overlooked in the hormone conversation. Together, these three macronutrients form the foundation of a metabolism that works with you instead of against you.

You'll learn why healthy fats help build hormones, why protein becomes more important with every passing decade, and why fiber is essential not just for digestion but also for detox, mood, and fat loss. We'll look at what actually happens to your metabolism after 40, and how to build your meals in a way that supports your energy, sleep, and cravings.

Forget food fear. It's time for food wisdom.

1: What Happens to Metabolism After 40

Something changes after 40. It's not just your body, it's the rules. What used to "work" in your thirties suddenly stops delivering the same results. You eat less, move more, and still the weight creeps on. You feel more tired after meals. You may notice bloating, mood swings, or sleep issues that weren't there before. This isn't about willpower or bad habits. It's about biology. Specifically, hormones.

Your metabolism is not just a calorie-burning machine. It's a complex conversation between your brain, gut, liver, hormones, and muscles. And when your hormones shift in midlife, the tone of that conversation changes. Sometimes it becomes quieter. Sometimes more chaotic. But either way, your body starts responding to food and stress in ways that feel unfamiliar.

Let's break down what's really happening beneath the surface.

Estrogen and Fat Storage

One of the most noticeable shifts is the loss of estrogen. As this hormone declines, your body becomes more prone to storing fat, especially around the abdomen. This isn't just cosmetic. Belly fat, or visceral fat, is metabolically active. It releases inflammatory signals that affect everything from blood sugar to mood to immune function.

Estrogen also played a protective role in keeping your metabolism flexible. It helped regulate how your body used glucose and fat for fuel. Without it, insulin resistance becomes more likely, and your ability to burn fat as energy decreases.

Insulin Resistance and Energy Drain

Insulin is the hormone responsible for shuttling glucose from your bloodstream into your cells. But after 40, especially in women, cells can become less responsive to insulin. This means glucose stays in your blood longer, triggering more insulin to be released. Over time, this process not only contributes to fat gain, but also leaves you feeling drained and foggy.

The more insulin resistant your body becomes, the harder it is to lose weight, even if you're eating less. This is why so many women feel frustrated by "doing everything right" but seeing no change. It's not that the rules don't apply. It's that the rules have changed.

Cortisol and the Midlife Stress Spiral

Cortisol, your stress hormone, becomes louder in midlife. Even if your life isn't more stressful, your body often perceives it that way. Declining estrogen reduces your resilience to stress, and everyday events like poor sleep, skipped meals, a tense conversation can cause exaggerated cortisol spikes.

High cortisol levels do several things. They raise blood sugar. They increase cravings, especially for sugar and salt. And they promote fat storage, particularly in the abdominal region. Cortisol also interferes with sleep, which then disrupts hunger hormones like ghrelin and leptin. It's a vicious loop that feeds on itself unless you intervene through nourishment and rhythm.

Muscle Loss and Metabolic Slowdown

Muscle is metabolically active tissue. It burns calories even at rest. But as you age, you naturally lose muscle unless you actively work to preserve or rebuild it. This loss of lean mass contributes to a slower metabolism and lower calorie needs overall. But it also affects strength, balance, and confidence in your own body.

Without enough protein and strength-building activity, you lose the very foundation that supports metabolic flexibility. More fat accumulates. Muscle dwindles. Energy drops. And the cycle continues unless you intentionally support your body with the right foods and movement.

The Role of Inflammation

Behind the scenes, chronic low-grade inflammation begins to rise with age. This isn't just about swollen joints or allergies. Inflammation is a silent disruptor of hormones. It contributes to insulin resistance, worsens cortisol spikes, and interferes with the way your body detoxes estrogen.

Many women don't realize that persistent bloating, brain fog, stubborn weight, and fatigue are not just symptoms but signs of inflammation. And food is one of the most powerful tools you have to calm it.

What This Means for You

> Forget calorie counting and cutting fat. Focus on building meals that communicate safety, nourishment, and stability to your system.

The takeaway is not that your body is broken. It's that your body is wise. It's adapting to a new hormonal landscape. And if you want to support it, you need to shift your strategy.

You need fat to make hormones. You need protein to rebuild tissue and prevent insulin spikes. You need fiber to escort toxins and excess estrogen out of your body.

These changes are not punishments. They are invitations to work with your body in a deeper, more informed way.

2: Rethinking Fat as Friend, Not Foe

The word "fat" has carried a heavy burden. For years, it was seen as something to avoid, reduce, or eliminate. "Low-fat" and "fat-free" labels once gave us a sense of control and virtue. But now we know better. Science, experience, and thousands of women's stories all point to one truth: fat is not the enemy. It never was.

In fact, fat plays an essential role in healing, hormone balance, weight loss, and long-term wellness, especially after 40. The problem wasn't fat. It was misinformation and fear.

Let's explore what fat really does in your body, which fats support healing, and how to bring them back into your meals with confidence.

Why Your Body Needs Fat

Fat is not just a fuel source. It is the raw material your body uses to build hormones like estrogen, progesterone, and testosterone. Without adequate fat, your endocrine system cannot function properly. You may experience irregular periods, worsened hot flashes, low libido, and mood instability, not because of aging alone, but because your body doesn't have what it needs to restore balance.

Fat also provides a cushion for your cells, protects your organs, helps you absorb vitamins A, D, E, and K, and keeps your skin, brain, and nerves functioning smoothly. It slows down digestion, which helps you feel full longer, and prevents the blood sugar spikes and crashes that lead to cravings and irritability.

In short, fat is fuel, structure, and communication. Your body understands it and depends on it.

The Types of Fat: Which to Embrace, Which to Avoid

Not all fats are created equal. The type of fat you eat can either support your hormones or trigger inflammation. Here's how to break it down:

1. Healthy Fats (Eat Daily)

- Monounsaturated fats: Found in olive oil, avocados, almonds, and macadamia nuts. These fats are anti-inflammatory, heart-friendly, and help regulate insulin.
- Omega-3 fatty acids: Found in fatty fish (like salmon, sardines, and mackerel), flaxseeds, chia seeds, and walnuts. These help reduce inflammation, balance mood, and protect brain health.
- Medium-chain triglycerides (MCTs): Found in coconut oil. Easily absorbed and converted into energy without requiring insulin spikes.
- Pasture-raised animal fats: In moderation, high-quality animal fats from organic or grass-fed sources can be nutrient-dense and stabilizing.

2. Inflammatory Fats (Minimize or Eliminate)

- Trans fats: Found in processed snacks, margarine, baked goods, and some restaurant fryers. These promote systemic inflammation and are linked to heart disease.

- Refined seed oils: Including soybean, corn, sunflower, safflower, and canola oil. These are high in omega-6 fatty acids, which in excess contribute to hormonal imbalance and joint inflammation.

Look beyond the front of the package. Read the ingredients list. If you see hydrogenated oils, shortenings, or vague "vegetable oil," put it back. Your hormones deserve better.

How Fat Supports Hormone Balance and Fat Loss

It may sound counterintuitive, but eating more healthy fat can actually help you lose body fat. That's because dietary fat does not spike insulin. When you eat a fat-rich meal, especially when paired with fiber and protein, your blood sugar remains stable. This reduces insulin secretion, which in turn helps unlock fat-burning pathways.

Fat also signals satiety more effectively than carbs or sugar. You feel fuller, longer, and you're less likely to overeat or snack impulsively. This improves cortisol levels by reducing the stress your body experiences from blood sugar crashes and food insecurity.

Many women find that once they start adding olive oil to their salads, avocado to their breakfast, and fatty fish to their dinners, their cravings drop dramatically. They stop chasing energy in the form of caffeine or sugar and begin feeling more grounded and satisfied.

Let Go of the "Low-Fat" Legacy

If you were raised in the era of low-fat everything, this shift can feel unfamiliar. You might still catch yourself measuring peanut butter with guilt or scraping off the yolk from your eggs. That's okay. Changing decades of messaging takes time.

But the science is clear. Low-fat diets have not been shown to improve long-term health outcomes. They have not made us leaner, healthier, or happier. In many cases, they made us more dependent on sugar and starch, which fuel inflammation and metabolic dysfunction.

Now is the time to rewrite the script. Fat is not indulgent but foundational, a choice your body recognizes and thanks you for.

Easy Ways to Add More Healthy Fats

Here are practical ways to increase your healthy fat intake without overthinking it:

- Add half an avocado to your morning eggs or smoothie bowl
- Drizzle olive oil over roasted vegetables or use it as a dip for steamed greens
- Snack on a handful of almonds or walnuts between meals
- Use chia or flaxseeds in oatmeal or yogurt
- Choose fatty fish two to three times per week
- Cook with coconut oil or ghee for flavor and stability
- Make dressings and sauces with tahini, avocado oil, or nut butters

You don't need to drown your food in oil. Small, consistent servings of healthy fats throughout the day can transform how you feel and function.

3: The Power of Protein for Women Over 40

Protein often gets overlooked in women's health conversations, especially beyond the gym crowd. But if you're over 40 and focused on healing, hormone balance, and fat loss, protein needs to move to the top of your nutrition priority list. This macronutrient is not just about muscle—although that's a major benefit. It also plays a key role in blood sugar regulation, metabolism, detoxification, and even mood.

After 40, your body begins to lose lean muscle mass at a steady pace unless you take steps to preserve and rebuild it. And here's the truth: muscle is your metabolic engine. When you support it with the right amount of protein, everything from fat loss to energy to emotional resilience improves.

Why Protein Needs Go Up, Not Down, After 40

Most women consume too little protein without realizing it. And as we age, we need more, not less. That's because declining estrogen contributes to muscle breakdown, which lowers your metabolic rate. If you're not eating enough protein, your body has no choice but to pull from its own tissues. That means more fat, less muscle, and a slower, more sluggish metabolism.

Protein is also essential for hormone production and repair. Every time your body produces a hormone, heals a cell, or clears out a toxin, it relies on amino acids, protein's building blocks, to do the work. Without a steady supply, your body runs slower, recovers slower, and feels more tired overall.

Protein for Fat Loss and Craving Control

Unlike carbs and fats, protein has a uniquely high thermic effect. This means your body burns more calories just digesting it. That alone gives it an edge when it comes to sustainable fat loss.

But protein does more than fuel the metabolism. It helps you feel satisfied. A protein-rich breakfast, for example, can reduce cravings all day by stabilizing blood sugar and improving hunger hormone signaling. It also increases levels of leptin, the hormone that tells your brain you're full.

If you've ever eaten a carb-heavy meal and felt hungry an hour later, you've felt the downside of imbalance. Protein solves that. It grounds you. It provides the slow, steady fuel your body prefers over sugar spikes and crashes.

Best Protein Sources for Hormone Health

Not all proteins are created equal. When choosing sources, focus on quality and variety. Aim for foods that are rich in amino acids, low in additives, and easy for your body to digest and use.

Animal-based proteins:

- Wild-caught fish (salmon, sardines, mackerel)
- Pasture-raised poultry and turkey
- Grass-fed beef (in moderation)
- Organic eggs
- Bone broth (rich in collagen and gut-supportive nutrients)

Plant-based proteins:

- Lentils and beans (black, pinto, chickpeas, navy)
- Tofu and tempeh (choose organic and minimally processed)
- Quinoa (a complete plant protein)
- Hemp, chia, and flax seeds
- Nuts and nut butters (also a healthy fat source)

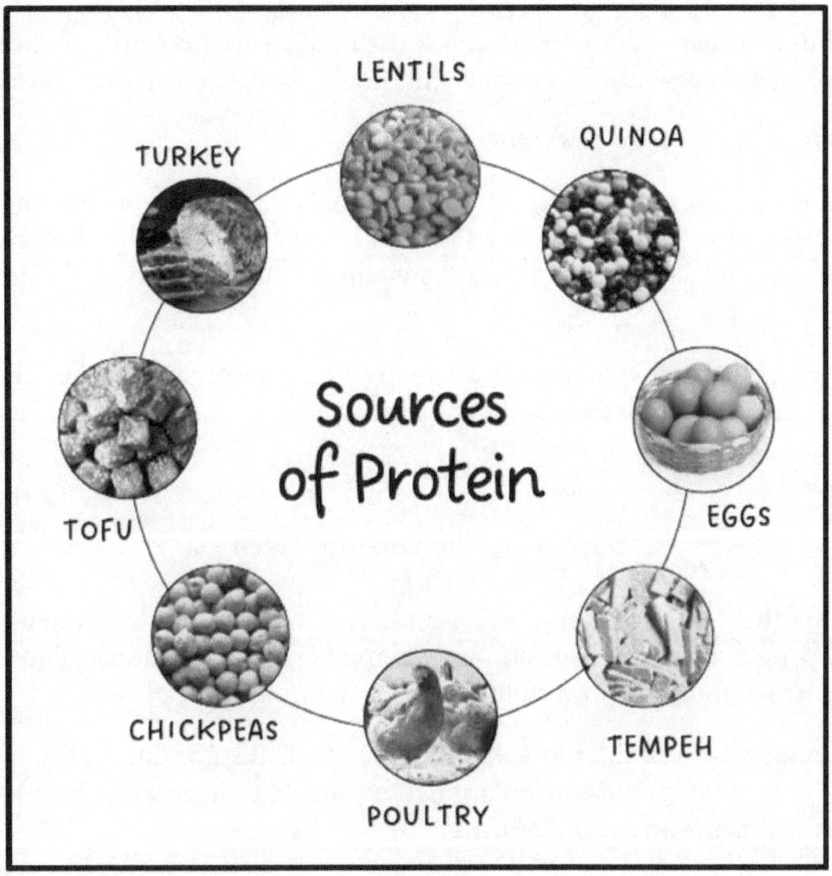

Balance is key. If you eat animal products, rotate them with plant-based sources to increase nutrient variety and fiber intake. And for plant-based eaters, combining foods like beans and rice can help provide the full range of amino acids your body needs.

How Much Protein Do You Actually Need?

There's no one-size-fits-all answer, but most women over 40 need significantly more than the standard recommendations. A helpful guideline is to aim for 0.8 to 1 gram of protein per pound of ideal body weight each day. So if your target weight is 140 pounds, you'd aim for about 110 to 140 grams of protein daily.

That may sound like a lot at first, but once you spread it out across meals and snacks, it becomes manageable. For example:

- Breakfast: 2 eggs + chia pudding (20–25 grams)
- Lunch: Grilled chicken salad with seeds and tahini dressing (30 grams)
- Snack: Protein smoothie with collagen or hemp protein (25 grams)

- Dinner: Salmon with lentils and greens (30–35 grams)

Eating protein consistently throughout the day is better than saving it all for dinner. Your body uses it more efficiently, and your energy stays steady.

When Protein Needs Extra Support

If you find it hard to meet your protein needs through food alone, clean protein powders can be a helpful tool. Look for options that are free from artificial sweeteners and unnecessary fillers. Whey protein isolate, collagen peptides, and plant-based blends (like pea and rice) are all great choices depending on your dietary needs.

Use smoothies to bridge the gap on busy mornings, or stir collagen into your coffee for a simple upgrade. Just remember, supplements are meant to supplement, not replace, whole food sources.

Building a Stronger, Leaner, More Resilient You

Adding more protein to your diet doesn't just support your metabolism. It builds a foundation for everything else: balanced hormones, stronger bones, better sleep, and fewer mood swings. It also helps you feel more satisfied and confident at the table, which makes the whole journey feel less like a struggle and more like self-respect in action.

This is not about turning into a bodybuilder. It's about becoming a woman who feeds herself well, owns her health, and no longer feels like her body is betraying her.

4: Fiber, The Unsung Hero

Fiber rarely gets the spotlight. It's not flashy. It doesn't have a trendy label. And it doesn't show up in social media posts the way protein or healthy fats do. But when it comes to hormone balance, fat loss, and long-term healing, fiber is one of the most powerful tools you can put on your plate.

For women over 40, fiber is more than just digestion support. It's a multitasking nutrient that touches nearly every system in your body. It calms inflammation, regulates hormones, balances blood sugar, and feeds the gut bacteria that help you detox and thrive.

Let's look closer at what fiber actually does, where to find it, and how to add more of it without turning your meals into a bland pile of plants.

What Is Fiber, Really?

Fiber is a type of carbohydrate that your body cannot fully digest. That might sound like a bad thing, but it's actually what makes it so helpful. Because fiber moves slowly through your digestive tract without being broken down into sugar, it helps regulate blood sugar levels, increase fullness, and keep your digestive system humming.

There are two main types:

- **Soluble fiber**, which dissolves in water and becomes gel-like. It helps lower cholesterol and stabilize blood sugar.
- **Insoluble fiber,** which adds bulk to your stool and supports regular bowel movements.

Most fiber-rich foods contain a mix of both types, and your body needs them equally.

How Fiber Supports Hormones and Fat Loss

> Fiber may be quiet, but it is one of your most powerful allies in hormone balance and long-term healing.

One of fiber's most overlooked roles is how it supports hormone clearance. Your body detoxes used-up estrogen through your liver and digestive tract. But if you're not eliminating regularly or you're low on fiber, that estrogen can recirculate. This contributes to estrogen dominance, a common hormonal imbalance that leads to bloating, weight gain, breast tenderness, and mood swings.

Fiber also feeds the good bacteria in your gut. These bacteria help produce short-chain fatty acids that reduce inflammation and support your immune system. A balanced gut microbiome improves mood, mental clarity, and even sleep, areas that often become unpredictable during perimenopause and menopause.

And let's not forget fat loss. High-fiber meals slow down digestion and help you feel full for longer. That means fewer spikes in insulin, fewer crashes, and fewer cravings. When your blood sugar stays steady, your body can access stored fat more easily, and your energy becomes smoother throughout the day.

Best Fiber-Rich Foods to Add Now

You don't need supplements to increase your fiber intake. Real food works better, tastes better, and comes with added benefits like antioxidants, minerals, and hydration.

Here are some of the best sources:

Vegetables:

- Broccoli, cauliflower, and Brussels sprouts
- Carrots, beets, and sweet potatoes
- Kale, spinach, collard greens, and arugula
- Artichokes, leeks, and zucchini

Fruits:

- Berries (especially raspberries and blackberries)
- Apples and pears (with skin)
- Avocado
- Oranges and kiwi

Legumes:

- Lentils and chickpeas
- Black beans, navy beans, and pinto beans
- Split peas

Whole grains:

- Quinoa
- Steel-cut oats
- Brown rice and wild rice
- Millet and buckwheat

Seeds and extras:

- Chia seeds
- Ground flaxseed
- Psyllium husk
- Almonds, walnuts, and pistachios

Aim for 25 to 35 grams of fiber per day. Most women get less than half of that, which leaves the gut undernourished and hormones unsupported.

How to Increase Fiber Without Bloating

One common mistake is going from low fiber to high fiber overnight. This can lead to bloating, gas, and digestive discomfort. The solution is to go slowly and hydrate well. Water is essential to help fiber move through your system.

Start by adding one fiber-rich food per meal. For example:

- Add chia seeds to your smoothie or yogurt
- Swap white rice for quinoa or lentils
- Include a leafy green salad before dinner
- Snack on berries or an apple with skin instead of crackers

Listen to your body as you increase fiber. Some adjustment is normal, but if discomfort persists, reduce slightly and add more cooked vegetables instead of raw until your system adapts.

The Gut–Hormone–Fiber Connection

Think of your gut as the command center for your hormonal health. If your gut is inflamed, sluggish, or lacking good bacteria, everything downstream gets affected. This includes cortisol regulation, estrogen detox, immune response, and nutrient absorption.

Fiber acts as a stabilizer. It gives your gut the tools to do its job well. It also binds to excess estrogen and toxins in the digestive tract, ensuring they leave the body rather than building up and causing problems.

By simply increasing fiber, many women notice less bloating, more regular digestion, reduced PMS symptoms, and more stable moods.

5: Creating a Macro-Balanced Plate

Once you understand the power of fat, fiber, and protein, the next question is usually: how do I pull this together on a plate? You don't need to count every gram or obsess over percentages. You just need to know how to visually balance your meals in a way that supports your hormones, metabolism, and long-term energy.

This is where the macro-balanced plate method becomes a game changer. It helps you build meals that keep blood sugar stable, reduce inflammation, and satisfy you both physically and emotionally.

Let's break down what a hormone-supportive plate looks like and how to make it work in real life.

What Is a Macro-Balanced Plate?

A macro-balanced plate contains all three key macronutrients, fat, protein, and fiber-rich carbohydrates, in portions that your body understands and responds to with stability, not stress.

Here's a simple visual:

- Half your plate: Non-starchy vegetables. These provide fiber, antioxidants, water, and bulk to your meal.
- One quarter of your plate: Lean protein. This gives your body the building blocks it needs to repair tissues and regulate hunger.
- One quarter of your plate: Healthy fats and complex carbs. Think avocado, olive oil, lentils, quinoa, or sweet potato.

You can also think in terms of food groups instead of strict measurements. The goal is to include a healthy fat, a high-quality protein, and at least one fiber-rich vegetable or legume at every meal.

Why Balance Matters After 40

Your body becomes more sensitive to blood sugar changes in midlife. Large spikes and crashes can trigger cortisol, worsen inflammation, and lead to more fat storage, especially around the belly. A macro-balanced plate reduces those swings by slowing digestion and providing a steady stream of energy.

It also prevents the late-night cravings and emotional eating that come when meals are too carb-heavy or too low in protein. When your body feels nourished, your mind feels calm.

Eating this way isn't restrictive. It's stabilizing. It tells your body it is safe, fed, and supported.

Sample Plate Templates for Each Meal

To help make this practical, here are ideas for breakfast, lunch, dinner, and snacks using the macro-balanced approach:

Breakfast

- Scrambled eggs cooked in olive oil
- Sautéed spinach and mushrooms
- Half an avocado or a side of berries with chia seeds

Lunch

- Grilled chicken or salmon
- Roasted sweet potatoes or quinoa
- Arugula and kale salad with olive oil and lemon dressing

Dinner

- Lentil and vegetable stew with turmeric and garlic
- Side of sautéed greens with walnuts
- Optional: a slice of baked acorn squash

Snack

- Greek yogurt with flaxseed and a handful of berries
- Hummus with sliced cucumber and bell peppers
- Boiled egg with a few almonds

You don't need to aim for perfection. Just build the habit of asking: do I have a source of protein, healthy fat, and fiber on my plate? If the answer is yes, you're already on the right track.

Tips for Making Macro-Balanced Eating Easier

1. Prep proteins ahead of time: Grill chicken, boil eggs, roast salmon, or make lentil patties in batches. Store them in the fridge for easy access.

2. Keep go-to fats stocked: Olive oil, avocados, nuts, seeds, tahini, and nut butters make it easy to add richness and nutrients in seconds.

3. Use frozen veggies: They're picked at peak ripeness and retain nutrients. Toss them into soups, sautés, or smoothies when fresh options are low.

4. Build bowls: Grain bowls, salad bowls, and soup bowls are all easy ways to mix and match proteins, fats, and vegetables without overcomplicating things.

5. Snack intentionally: Avoid going carb-only. Pair a fruit with nuts, or veggies with hummus to keep your blood sugar stable between meals.

Consistency matters more than novelty. You don't need a Pinterest-perfect plate every time. You just need balance and intention.

What About Carbs?

Carbohydrates are not the enemy. But the type and timing of carbs matter more as your hormones shift. Fiber-rich carbs like lentils, oats, quinoa, root vegetables, and beans provide lasting energy and support gut health. Highly refined carbs like white bread, pastries, and sweetened snacks can spike insulin and derail your progress.

If you love carbs, there's room for them. Just choose slower-burning, high-fiber options and pair them with protein and fat. This keeps blood sugar steady and reduces the crash-and-crave cycle.

You don't need to eliminate any food group completely. Just prioritize whole, unprocessed sources that give you more than they take.

A Plate That Works With You, Not Against You

The beauty of this approach is how sustainable it feels. It doesn't require a scale, an app, or a spreadsheet. It simply asks you to check in with your plate and give your body what it actually needs.

You'll begin to notice that meals are more satisfying. You'll feel less bloated. Your cravings will fade. And perhaps most importantly, you'll feel a sense of peace and partnership with your body again.

6: Real-Life Challenges and How to Adjust

Even with the best intentions, real life has a way of testing your new habits. You might be excited about macro-balanced meals and hormone-friendly choices, but then the week gets hectic, your fridge goes empty, or you're eating dinner at a friend's house with zero control over the menu.

Don't worry. These situations are not roadblocks. They are just opportunities to practice flexibility. Healing is not about perfection. It's about learning how to adjust, bounce back, and keep showing up for yourself.

Eating Out or Traveling

When you're away from your own kitchen, focus on the basics. Look for meals that include a clean protein, non-starchy vegetables, and a healthy fat. Grilled fish with vegetables. A chicken salad with olive oil dressing. A burrito bowl without the tortilla.

Ask for swaps without guilt. Most restaurants are happy to sub fries for a side salad or steamed vegetables. Traveling? Pack a few essentials like almonds, protein bars, or nut butter packets. They can bridge the gap when you're stuck in a car, airport, or conference room without great options.

Feeling Stuck or Hitting a Plateau

Sometimes your progress slows, and it feels like nothing is working. Instead of overcorrecting, pause and reassess. Are you eating enough protein? Are your meals still fiber-rich and satisfying? Are you hydrating, moving your body, and getting enough sleep?

Sometimes the issue isn't your food but stress, hormones, or a lack of rhythm. Get back to your foundation. Simple meals. Gentle movement. Solid sleep. Then adjust your portions, protein variety, or timing if needed.

Small shifts often unlock big changes.

Making It Work With a Family or Budget

You don't have to cook separate meals for everyone. Use the macro-balanced plate method to build a flexible base, then let each family member customize. You might eat your taco filling over a bed of greens while others use tortillas. You might skip the sugary sauce but enjoy the protein and roasted vegetables with everyone else.

Budget-friendly proteins like eggs, canned salmon, beans, and lentils can stretch across multiple meals. Frozen vegetables are just as nutritious as fresh and last longer. Healing meals don't need fancy ingredients, just some thoughtful balance.

What matters most is that you keep showing up for your health. Even on the messy days. Especially on the messy days.

You've just unlearned decades of noise and reconnected with something simple and powerful: your body's deep wisdom.

You now understand that fat is not the villain. It's the builder of hormones, the stabilizer of mood, and the keeper of satiety. That protein is not just for athletes. It's the structure that keeps your energy up, your metabolism strong, and your hunger calm. That fiber is not a bland afterthought. It's a quiet force that clears toxins, feeds your gut, and makes hormone balance possible.

These three macronutrients are not trendy. They are timeless. Your body has always needed them. The difference now is that you are choosing them with purpose.

In the next chapter, we'll take these ideas and shape them into a personalized plan that fits your life, your rhythms, and your goals. You'll learn how to build your week, stock your kitchen, and bring balance into even the busiest days.

PART THREE: YOUR PERSONALIZED PLAN

CHAPTER 7: WHAT TO EAT AND WHY IT WORKS

You've learned a lot. You now understand how your hormones shift after 40, why your metabolism feels different, and how macronutrients like fat, protein, and fiber can support healing and balance. This knowledge is powerful, but now it's time to turn it into nourishment.

Information alone won't reset your hormones. What changes your body is what you do with that information every day, every week, and every time you step into your kitchen. This chapter is about making that shift, from theory to practice, from rules to rhythm.

This is not a strict meal plan. It's not a cleanse or challenge or countdown. Instead, you'll learn how to choose foods that love your hormones, reduce inflammation, support digestion, and help you feel full and calm without needing to count, track, or stress.

When food becomes less about restriction and more about communication, everything changes. You begin to see your meals not as something to fear or fix, but as a way of sending clear, supportive messages to your body. You say: here's energy. Here's nourishment. Here's what you need to function, heal, and thrive.

This chapter will guide you through the Galveston Diet food framework, how it works, how to apply it, and why it's flexible enough to fit real life. You'll learn what foods to emphasize, how to portion without obsessing, how to time your meals in a way that supports fat loss and hormone rhythm, and how to build consistency without burnout.

You don't need to be perfect. You need to be supported. That's what this chapter is here to do.

1: The Galveston Diet Food Philosophy

If you've ever felt like food rules keep changing—low-carb, low-fat, plant-based, paleo, intermittent fasting, keto—it's because diet culture thrives on confusion. But real healing doesn't come from trendy extremes. It comes from understanding how your body works and feeding it accordingly.

The Galveston Diet is not a trend. It's a way of eating rooted in science, designed specifically for the hormonal shifts that happen after 40. It's anti-inflammatory, high in fiber and healthy fats, and rich in protein to support muscle, mood, and metabolism. It's built for women in midlife, but it's flexible enough for every season of life.

Let's walk through what makes this approach different and why it works.

Food as Support, Not Suppression

Traditional diets are often about suppressing hunger, shrinking the body, and following rigid rules. But your body after 40 needs more support, not less. The Galveston Diet uses food to send the right signals—calm down inflammation, stabilize insulin, reduce cortisol, and clear out excess estrogen.

This isn't about forcing your body into submission. It's about helping your body feel safe and strong enough to do what it was designed to do.

Nutrient Density Over Calorie Control

Calories are not meaningless, but they're not the full story. Two meals with the same calorie count can have completely different effects on your hormones. A sugary granola bar may trigger blood sugar spikes, cravings, and fatigue, while a hard-boiled egg with avocado slices helps you feel grounded, satisfied, and focused for hours.

The Galveston approach prioritizes nutrient density, with foods that give you the most vitamins, minerals, fiber, healthy fats, and antioxidants per bite. This naturally reduces overeating because your body feels nourished, not deprived.

When you feed your cells well, they perform better. Your skin glows. Your energy steadies. Your cravings fade. It's not about eating less. It's about eating better.

Food as Hormonal Messenger

Every food you eat sends a message to your endocrine system. Will this meal raise blood sugar? Will it spike cortisol? Will it slow digestion or cause inflammation? Your body listens and responds, even when you're not paying attention.

That's why the Galveston Diet focuses on ingredients that help regulate insulin, support gut health, promote estrogen detox, and reduce inflammation. We're not just talking about nutrition. We're talking about communication.

Examples:

- Fiber-rich vegetables help clear out excess estrogen
- Omega-3 fats calm your nervous system and lower cortisol
- Protein increases satiety and supports lean muscle
- Fermented foods promote a healthy gut microbiome

These effects are real. And when you stack them together, meal after meal, the body starts to respond in powerful ways.

Built-In Flexibility, Not Perfection

One of the most important parts of this approach is that it's forgiving. There are no gold stars for getting it perfect. There is no punishment for missing a day.

> The goal is consistency over time,
> not immediate transformation.

You will have travel days, family gatherings, busy weeks, and moments of "I just need something quick." That's okay. The Galveston framework teaches you how to pivot with purpose. Maybe it's choosing the protein and veggie option on a menu. Maybe it's packing almonds and dried lentil snacks for a flight. Maybe it's skipping the drive-through fries but enjoying a small glass of red wine at dinner.

You don't fail when you stray. You reset with the next bite.

For Every Kind of Eater

Whether you're an omnivore, vegetarian, or mostly plant-based, this philosophy can work for you. It's not about one perfect style. It's about emphasizing foods that lower inflammation, feed your gut, balance your hormones, and leave you feeling steady and nourished.

You can tailor it based on your culture, preferences, health goals, and season of life. It's a framework, not a formula.

Real Food Over Products

Another key distinction: the Galveston Diet prioritizes real, whole foods over packaged health products. While supplements and protein powders can play a supporting role, your foundation should be built on simple, recognizable ingredients, like vegetables, fish, nuts, seeds, legumes, fruits, and healthy oils.

This approach helps lower your toxic load, support detoxification, and reduce hidden inflammation from food additives, artificial sweeteners, and preservatives.

Whole food is always the starting point. Healing begins at the grocery cart.

2: How Food Timing Affects Hormones

What you eat matters, but when you eat can be just as important, especially after 40. Your hormones respond not only to what's on your plate but also to the rhythm of your meals. Skipping meals, eating late at night, or grazing all day can throw off your body's natural cycles, raise cortisol, and prevent fat loss, even if your food choices are clean.

Food is information, and timing is the tone in which that message is delivered. A nourishing meal eaten in the right window can calm your body and signal healing. The same meal eaten at midnight, under stress, or after a full day of blood sugar roller coasters, may land very differently.

This is where timed eating enters the picture, not as a strict fasting regime, but as a way to bring rhythm and predictability to your hormones.

The Hormonal Flow of the Day

Your hormones follow a daily pattern called your circadian rhythm. Cortisol is highest in the morning to help you wake up and get moving. Insulin sensitivity also peaks earlier in the day, meaning your body processes carbs more efficiently at breakfast and lunch than at dinner.

Melatonin, your sleep hormone, rises in the evening, signaling rest and repair. Late-night eating disrupts this pattern. When you eat too close to bedtime, your body is forced to digest instead of restore. This can affect sleep quality, increase overnight cortisol, and interfere with hormone detoxification.

Timed eating aligns your meals with your internal clock. It gives your digestive system time to rest, your hormones space to rebalance, and your body the chance to burn fat rather than constantly process incoming food.

What Is Timed Eating?

Timed eating is a flexible approach to meal spacing, often using a daily eating window, like 10am to 6pm or 11am to 7pm. During that window, you eat your meals and snacks. Outside that window, you rest and hydrate.

This gives your body a fasting window of about 14 to 16 hours overnight, which has been shown to support blood sugar regulation, reduce inflammation, and improve metabolic markers.

Timed eating is not about starving yourself or skipping breakfast just to "fit the window." It's about creating a consistent rhythm that honors your hormones.

Benefits of Eating in a Set Window

- Stabilized blood sugar: When meals are spaced predictably, your body gets better at regulating insulin and burning fat.
- Lower cortisol levels: Predictable meal timing reduces food-related stress and lowers the need for cortisol spikes.
- Improved digestion: The gut functions best when it has time to fully digest before the next meal.
- Reduced inflammation: Timed eating allows your body to enter a repair phase during fasting hours.
- Better sleep: Avoiding food too close to bedtime supports melatonin production and hormonal detox.

How to Choose a Window That Works

You don't have to force yourself into a rigid schedule. Start with a 12-hour fast, maybe from 7pm to 7am, and build from there as it feels natural. The most common windows are:

- 12:12 – Eat from 8am to 8pm
- 14:10 – Eat from 10am to 8pm
- 16:8 – Eat from 11am to 7pm

The key is consistency. Your body thrives on routine. Eating your first meal at a similar time each day helps regulate hunger hormones like ghrelin and leptin, which support satiety and reduce emotional eating.

What to Break Your Fast With

How you break your fast matters. After a long stretch without food, your body is especially sensitive to what you eat first. A sugary pastry or juice bomb can spike insulin and derail your day before it starts.

Instead, choose meals rich in protein, fiber, and healthy fat. Examples:

- Scrambled eggs with avocado and sautéed spinach
- Chia pudding with almond butter and berries
- Smoothie with collagen, flaxseed, frozen berries, and almond milk

These meals support stable energy, reduce cravings, and set a steady tone for your blood sugar curve.

Adapting If Timed Eating Feels Challenging

If you've had a history of disordered eating or feel anxious about skipping breakfast, don't pressure yourself into a fasting window. You can still honor your hormones with regular meals spaced about four to five hours apart. Just avoid grazing all day, and give your digestive system at least a 12-hour overnight break.

The goal is to reduce the frequency and chaos of eating, not to deprive yourself.

Food Timing Is Hormonal Communication

When you eat at consistent times, your body relaxes. It stops constantly scanning for energy and starts trusting that fuel will come. That trust creates hormonal stability. Cravings quiet down. Your metabolism becomes more efficient. Your energy lasts longer.

This is not about skipping meals to lose weight. It's about giving your body a break so it can heal and reset.

3: Portioning with Purpose

After years of dieting, many women associate portion control with restriction, hunger, and measuring every bite. But in the context of healing and hormone balance, portioning isn't about shrinking your meals, it's about targeting your nourishment. It's about giving your body enough of what it actually needs to function at its best.

The Galveston Diet approach is about getting the right types of food in the right proportions to stabilize blood sugar, reduce inflammation, and support metabolic repair. The best part? You can do this visually, no tracking apps required.

When you learn to build your meals using portioning principles that support your hormones, your body responds. Energy improves. Cravings decrease. Fat loss becomes easier. Your meals become a tool for healing, not a source of anxiety.

Why Portioning Matters After 40

In midlife, your body's response to food becomes more sensitive. The same oversized plate of pasta that once left you feeling fine may now lead to bloating, fatigue, or a sugar crash. That's because your insulin sensitivity has likely declined, your estrogen levels have shifted, and your muscle mass may be lower.

Eating with intention helps correct this. It prevents overloading your system with one macronutrient (like carbs), while ensuring you get enough of the others (like protein and fat) that support stable blood sugar, hormone detox, and lean muscle maintenance.

This isn't about tiny meals. It's about balanced ones.

The Galveston Plate Proportions

Here's a simple visual guideline to follow for most meals:

- Half of your plate: Non-starchy vegetables (like leafy greens, cauliflower, zucchini, bell peppers, cucumbers, broccoli)

- One quarter: Protein (such as salmon, chicken, lentils, tofu, eggs)
- One quarter: Healthy fats and complex carbs (avocado, olive oil, nuts, quinoa, sweet potato, lentils)

You can also think in terms of components rather than plate space:

- Protein: Aim for 20 to 30 grams per meal
- Healthy fat: Include 1 to 2 tablespoons of oil or 1 small portion of nuts, seeds, or avocado
- Fiber-rich carbs: Choose whole sources like lentils, vegetables, berries, or quinoa

When in doubt, ask: Do I have something to stabilize blood sugar (protein), something to support hormones and fullness (fat), and something to fuel digestion and detox (fiber)?

Adjusting for Body Type and Activity

Portion sizes are not one-size-fits-all. You can use the plate method as a starting point and adjust based on how you feel. If you are highly active, nursing, or recovering from illness, you may need slightly larger portions of protein or complex carbs. If you're feeling sluggish, bloated, or inflamed, you may benefit from dialing up the veggies and dialing down the starches temporarily.

Listen to your body. Signs that you may need to increase protein or fat:

- Crashing energy two hours after a meal
- Feeling hungry again too quickly
- Intense evening cravings
- Muscle loss or weakness despite exercise

Signs you may be overdoing a particular macro:

- Feeling heavy or sluggish after meals
- Bloating or slow digestion
- Afternoon fatigue or sugar crashes
- Trouble sleeping after high-carb dinners

Let your body guide you, not the scale or a diet app.

Common Mistakes in Portioning

- 1. Skimping on protein

Women often under-eat protein, especially at breakfast. A single egg only provides about 6 grams. You likely need two to three times that to feel full and stay energized.

- 2. Overloading healthy fats

While fats are essential, it's easy to turn a meal into a calorie bomb by adding too many oils, nuts, or seeds.

Stick to one or two sources per meal.

- 3. Treating fruit like a free food

Fruits are healthy, but they're still a form of sugar. Use them as part of a balanced plate, not the main event.

- 4. Forgetting fiber

Fiber slows digestion, feeds your gut, and supports hormone clearance. Without it, even a high-protein meal can leave you unbalanced.

- 5. Grazing all day

Even healthy snacks can disrupt your hormone rhythm if they're constant. Focus on full meals spaced a few hours apart.

Realistic Portioning Examples

Breakfast:

- 2 scrambled eggs (12g protein)
- Sautéed kale and mushrooms (fiber and antioxidants)
- Half an avocado (healthy fat)
- Side of berries (light carbs and antioxidants)

Lunch:

- Grilled chicken breast (30g protein)
- Roasted Brussels sprouts and red peppers
- Quinoa with olive oil drizzle
- Herbal tea or water with lemon

Dinner:

- Lentil and veggie stew (fiber, protein, and carbs)
- Side of sautéed spinach with garlic
- Sprinkle of pumpkin seeds for crunch and zinc
- Optional: baked sweet potato if needed for extra energy

Use your plate as a canvas. You don't need to be exact. Just be intentional.

4: Food Lists That Heal, Not Harm

Knowing what to eat gets a lot easier when you have a framework to guide your choices. The Galveston Diet isn't about strict food rules or cutting out everything you love. It's about building your meals around foods that lower inflammation, balance hormones, and support steady energy while reducing the ones that interfere with those goals.

Think of this approach as three tiers: Emphasize, Rotate, and Minimize. It's not a yes-or-no list. It's a support system. The more you build your meals around the "Emphasize" list, the more your body responds with clarity, strength, and balance.

These are foods that do more than fill you up. They help your body communicate, detox, and repair.

Emphasize: Eat These Often

These foods support hormone balance, fight inflammation, stabilize blood sugar, and nourish your gut. These should form the core of most meals.

Proteins:

- Wild-caught salmon, sardines, and mackerel
- Pasture-raised chicken and turkey
- Organic eggs
- Grass-fed beef (1–2 times per week)
- Lentils, chickpeas, black beans
- Tofu and tempeh (organic)

Fats:

- Extra virgin olive oil
- Avocados and avocado oil
- Chia, flax, hemp, and pumpkin seeds
- Walnuts, almonds, pistachios
- Ghee or grass-fed butter (in moderation)

Vegetables:

- Cruciferous: broccoli, cauliflower, Brussels sprouts
- Leafy greens: kale, spinach, chard, arugula
- Rainbow veggies: bell peppers, carrots, zucchini, beets
- Alliums: garlic, onions, leeks

Fruits (low glycemic):

- Berries: blueberries, raspberries, strawberries, blackberries
- Apples and pears (with skin)
- Pomegranate, kiwi, citrus fruits

Carbs (fiber-rich):

- Quinoa
- Steel-cut oats
- Sweet potatoes and other root vegetables
- Lentils and beans

Flavor and function:

- Fresh herbs: parsley, cilantro, rosemary, basil
- Spices: turmeric, ginger, cinnamon, cumin
- Fermented foods: sauerkraut, kimchi, kefir, plain Greek yogurt

Rotate: Eat These Sometimes

These foods can absolutely fit into a healing lifestyle, especially when prepared simply and eaten with intention. They're supportive but not essential every day.

Proteins:

- Goat cheese or sheep cheese (small amounts)
- Organic tofu and tempeh (alternate with legumes)
- Canned salmon or tuna (watch sodium and sourcing)

Fats:

- Nut butters (peanut, almond, cashew)
- Coconut oil and milk
- Sesame oil, sunflower seeds

Vegetables and starches:

- Cooked white potatoes
- Corn (organic, if possible)
- Butternut squash and acorn squash
- Peas, edamame

Grains:

- Brown rice and wild rice
- Millet, farro, barley (rotate if tolerated well)
- Sprouted grain bread or tortillas (minimally processed)

Fruits (moderate glycemic):

- Bananas
- Grapes, cherries, mango (small servings)
- Dried fruits (unsweetened and limited to small portions)

Minimize: Eat These Rarely

These foods tend to raise inflammation, spike insulin, irritate the gut, or interfere with hormone detoxification. You don't need to fear them, but reducing their presence in your weekly meals can significantly improve how you feel.

Highly processed foods:

- Packaged snacks (chips, crackers, granola bars)
- Breakfast cereals (especially with added sugar)
- Instant noodles or boxed meals
- Energy drinks, sweetened coffee beverages

Inflammatory fats:

- Soybean, corn, canola, and vegetable oil
- Hydrogenated oils and trans fats
- Margarine and shortening

Refined carbohydrates:

- White bread, white rice, regular pasta
- Baked goods: cookies, muffins, pastries
- Candy, sweetened yogurts, and ice cream

Beverages:

- Soda (regular and diet)
- Fruit juices (even 100 percent)
- Alcohol (especially more than 3–4 times per week)

Meats and dairy:

- Processed meats: bacon, sausage, deli meat

- Factory-farmed beef and poultry
- Conventional dairy (especially sweetened or flavored)

Grocery List Goals: Weekly Staples to Keep on Hand

Fridge:

- Eggs
- Leafy greens
- Cooked lentils or beans
- Leftover protein (grilled chicken, salmon)
- Chopped veggies in containers
- Berries and citrus

Freezer:

- Wild-caught fish
- Frozen broccoli, spinach, and green beans
- Cauliflower rice
- Frozen blueberries and mango
- Bone broth cubes or pouches

Pantry:

- Quinoa, oats, brown rice
- Olive oil, avocado oil
- Chia seeds, ground flaxseed
- Almonds, walnuts, pumpkin seeds
- Canned beans, tuna, and tomatoes
- Spices: turmeric, cinnamon, garlic powder

Having the right foods available makes it easier to build balanced meals without stress. If you prep your kitchen, your meals will follow.

5: Supportive Habits Around Food

Your meals don't exist in isolation. They are shaped by your stress levels, your sleep quality, your schedule, and even the way you breathe as you eat. Two women could eat the same bowl of food and have completely different responses depending on what's happening around and within them.

This is why supportive habits matter. They help your body receive nourishment more effectively. They reduce hormonal chaos and create the conditions for food to become fuel instead of friction.

Let's explore the practical habits that can take your hormone-healing meals to the next level.

Eating Without Multitasking

When you eat while scrolling, driving, or working, your body stays in a state of mild stress. This keeps you in sympathetic mode, your fight-or-flight state, rather than the parasympathetic mode, where digestion, absorption, and repair happen.

To shift into this healing state:

- Sit down at a table, not a desk or car seat
- Take three deep breaths before your first bite
- Chew slowly and intentionally
- Put your fork down between bites

These simple habits help activate your vagus nerve and support digestion from the top down. You'll not only absorb more nutrients, but also feel fuller and more satisfied without needing more food.

Spacing Out Meals

Constant snacking or grazing, even on healthy foods, keeps your insulin levels elevated. This prevents fat burning and can also exhaust your digestive system. Your body needs time between meals to fully digest and shift into a restorative state.

Aim for:

- 3 solid meals per day, each balanced with protein, fat, and fiber
- 4 to 5 hours between meals without grazing
- Optional snack only if needed for energy, activity, or blood sugar support

Let your body experience true hunger before your next meal. This strengthens metabolic flexibility and reduces insulin resistance over time.

Post-Meal Movement

One of the easiest and most effective habits for blood sugar regulation is moving after you eat. A 10 to 20 minute walk after meals lowers blood glucose, improves insulin sensitivity, and reduces that afternoon crash or evening craving.

You don't need a gym session. A walk around the block, a few minutes of light stretching, or even housework counts. It's not about burning calories. It's about telling your body, "We're using this fuel wisely."

Sleep, Stress, and Meal Timing

Your cortisol levels rise when you sleep poorly or stay in a constant state of tension. This has a direct effect on how your body handles food. When cortisol is elevated, you're more likely to store fat, experience cravings, and feel hungry even when your energy needs are met.

Here's how to support your hormones outside of mealtime:

- Prioritize 7 to 8 hours of quality sleep
- Create a wind-down routine in the evening (no food 2–3 hours before bed)
- Use stress management tools like breathwork, journaling, or meditation
- Avoid caffeine after noon if it affects your sleep

When stress is high, keep meals extra simple: broths, cooked vegetables, lean proteins, and easily digestible fats. Your gut and hormones will thank you.

Staying Hydrated the Right Way

Dehydration mimics hunger and fatigue. It also slows digestion and increases cortisol. But what you drink, and when, matters.

Supportive hydration habits:

- Start your morning with 12 to 16 ounces of water before coffee or food
- Sip water throughout the day, not all at once
- Add a pinch of sea salt or a squeeze of lemon for electrolyte balance
- Avoid drinking large amounts of water with meals (this dilutes stomach acid)
- Herbal teas like ginger, peppermint, or chamomile can aid digestion

Hydration is more than water. It's about helping your cells carry out the healing work you're setting in motion with your meals.

Creating a Ritual Around Eating

When you bring intention into your meals, your body responds. Instead of seeing food as a task or threat, it becomes a rhythm. A reset. A way to ground and center yourself.

Try this:

- Light a candle or put on calming music during meals
- Use real plates and utensils instead of containers
- Say a short word of gratitude before your first bite
- Pause halfway through to check in with how you feel

These small shifts create presence. And presence is where healing begins.

Food as Rhythm, Not Rules

You've just taken a major step forward. You now understand that healing your body is not about counting every bite, but about feeding yourself with awareness, rhythm, and purpose.

You've learned how to portion your meals in ways that support your hormones. You've discovered which foods help your body reset and which ones quietly disrupt your balance. You've seen how timing, stress, and even how you sit down to eat can affect the way your body processes every meal.

But most importantly, you've begun to rebuild trust with your body. You're learning to speak its language. And it's listening.

Balance your plate. Choose foods that support your hormones. Eat in a rhythm that gives your body rest and renewal. Tune in to how you feel after meals, not just how you look. These are the tools that turn nutrition into a sustainable lifestyle, not a cycle of control and crash.

In the next chapter, you'll take everything you've learned and translate it into real life. We'll build your weekly blueprint: meal planning, grocery lists, prep strategies, and the systems that make it all stick, even when life gets busy.

CHAPTER 8: BLUEPRINT FOR YOUR WEEK

Eating with intention feels great, until real life kicks in. A busy Monday. A skipped grocery run. A missed lunch that turns into an all-day blood sugar roller coaster. Even the most motivated woman can find herself reaching for whatever is easy, fast, or familiar, but not necessarily what supports healing.

That's why goals aren't enough. Healing through food doesn't happen by accident. It happens through systems.

You don't need another rule to follow. You need rhythms that support your hormones automatically. You need repeatable routines that reduce stress, simplify decision-making, and help you stay nourished, even when life gets messy.

This chapter is not about planning a perfect week. It's about designing a realistic one. A week where your meals feel doable, your kitchen works for you, and your food choices happen before the hunger or chaos hits. You'll learn how to plan your meals without micromanaging them, how to shop with purpose, and how to batch-prep your staples without spending your entire weekend in the kitchen.

You'll also learn how to build in flexibility. Because some weeks, you'll cook three full meals a day. Other weeks, you'll be leaning on broth, frozen salmon, and hard-boiled eggs. And both are valid. Systems aren't rigid. They're there to catch you when life pulls you away from your ideal.

Healing isn't just about food. It's about the environment around your food. When your fridge is stocked, your plan is simple, and your meals are halfway prepped, everything changes. You spend less time deciding and more time nourishing.

This chapter is your blueprint for that shift, from scattered to supported, from guessing to grounded. It's not about getting it right. It's about making it work.

1: The Weekly Rhythm—Your Hormone-Supportive Flow

Your body loves rhythm. Just like your heartbeat, breath, and sleep-wake cycle, your hormones operate on patterns. Estrogen, cortisol, insulin, and melatonin all follow a rhythm—daily, monthly, and seasonally. When you create weekly meal rhythms that match those patterns, your body feels safe, grounded, and ready to heal.

This isn't about rigid meal plans. It's about anchoring your week with simple, predictable habits that remove guesswork and lower hormonal stress. Structure doesn't mean you lose freedom. It means you gain clarity. When meals become part of your routine, your hormones learn to relax.

Let's break down what a hormone-supportive week can look like and how to make it your own.

Anchor Your Days with Predictable Meal Flow

Your hormones thrive on consistency. Start by anchoring your meals around three basic touchpoints:

- A protein-rich breakfast or first meal (depending on your eating window)
- A balanced midday meal with fiber and fat

- A lighter, anti-inflammatory dinner eaten at least 2–3 hours before bed

This structure supports cortisol's natural rise in the morning, keeps insulin stable throughout the day, and allows melatonin to rise properly at night.

Even if your schedule changes, aim to keep meal timing relatively steady. Your metabolism, digestion, and blood sugar regulation all benefit from rhythm.

Use "Meal Themes" to Simplify Your Week

The easiest way to reduce meal planning stress is to stop reinventing the wheel every week. Instead, create a simple template using themed days:

- Meatless Monday: lentil curry, black bean tacos, quinoa bowls
- Sheet-Pan Tuesday: salmon and veggies, chicken and sweet potato
- Soup & Salad Wednesday: veggie soup + arugula salad with nuts and avocado
- Slow Cooker Thursday: shredded chicken, bone broth stew, bean chili
- Flex Friday: leftovers, pantry staples, or a simple bowl dinner
- Social Saturday: dinner out or potluck-friendly meal
- Prep Sunday: light cooking + batch prep for the week

These themes aren't rules. They're rhythm-makers. They guide your grocery list, simplify decision-making, and allow room for flexibility.

Cycle Meals with Your Energy and Mood

Your hormone levels, energy, and cravings change throughout the week and even throughout the day. Build your food routine to support this ebb and flow.

- Early in the week:

You might feel more focused and motivated. Lean into clean, balanced meals and slightly lighter eating as your body resets from the weekend.

- Midweek:

Work and stress may peak. Add grounding meals like hearty soups, roasted root vegetables, and good fats to support cortisol regulation.

- Late week or weekends:

Cravings may show up, or social plans may pull you off track. Plan for flexibility. Have one or two easy fallback meals ready. Enjoy treats mindfully and return to balance without guilt.

You don't need to eat the same way every day. You need a pattern that flexes with your life and still keeps you nourished.

Include Rest and Reset Days

Food is only part of the rhythm. Recovery is the other side. Create space for lower-effort days in both your cooking and your expectations.

Rest days could include:

- Minimal cooking (leftovers, simple bowls, smoothies)
- Extra hydration and herbal teas
- Light movement (walks, stretching)
- Early dinners and longer overnight fasting windows

These gentle days help reset digestion, reduce cortisol, and give your nervous system a break. You don't always need to push. Sometimes healing comes from pause.

Sample Hormone-Supportive Week at a Glance

Monday:

- Chia pudding with berries
- Lentil veggie bowl
- Salmon with roasted cauliflower and tahini

Tuesday:

- Smoothie with collagen, spinach, flax
- Grilled chicken with arugula and quinoa
- Stuffed sweet potato with beans and avocado

Wednesday:

- Scrambled eggs with mushrooms
- Vegetable soup with pumpkin seeds
- Turkey meatballs and spaghetti squash

Thursday:

- Oats with chia and almond butter
- Leftover lentils and steamed greens
- Slow cooker chicken with root vegetables

Friday:

- Protein shake + nuts
- Hummus wrap with salad
- Dinner out or shrimp stir-fry at home

Saturday:

- Eggs and roasted veggies
- Leftovers or flexible bowl
- Social meal, mindful portions

Sunday:

- Simple breakfast or fast
- Big salad or soup
- Early dinner and prep for the week

2: How to Meal Plan Without Overwhelm

Meal planning doesn't have to feel like a second job. In fact, if it's leaving you overwhelmed, you're likely doing too much. You don't need a color-coded spreadsheet or 21 perfectly portioned meals stacked in plastic containers. You need a simple, flexible structure that gives you clarity, not pressure.

This section walks you through a hormone-supportive meal planning process that actually fits your life. It's designed to help you feel nourished, not managed.

Let's reframe meal planning into something doable, intuitive, and kind.

Step 1: Choose Your Core Proteins

Every good meal plan starts with your anchors. In this case, that means protein. Choose 2 or 3 proteins for the week that you can prep ahead or cook fresh depending on time.

Examples:

- Salmon and pasture-raised chicken
- Lentils and eggs
- Ground turkey and wild-caught shrimp
- Tofu and black beans

Once you've chosen your proteins, it becomes easier to build out your sides, veggies, and fats. These are the keystone of your hormone-balancing plate.

Step 2: Pick 4 to 5 Veggies to Rotate

Now build your plan around seasonal or favorite vegetables. These should be easy to prep, cook quickly, and pair well with your proteins. Try to include:

- One leafy green (like kale, arugula, or spinach)
- One cruciferous veggie (like broccoli, cabbage, or cauliflower)

- One starchy option (like sweet potato or squash)
- One colorful veggie (like bell peppers, zucchini, or carrots)
- One gut-supportive food (like onions, garlic, or leeks)

Prep them in advance or buy pre-cut versions if that makes it easier. Cook in big batches so you can mix and match throughout the week.

Step 3: Add Fats, Flavors, and Sides

This is where the variety and satisfaction come in. Keep it simple:

- Healthy fats: avocado, olive oil, nuts, seeds, tahini
- Carbs: quinoa, lentils, beans, steel-cut oats, root vegetables
- Flavors: lemon, fresh herbs, vinegars, mustard, coconut aminos, ginger, garlic, chili flakes

Build your grocery list from these categories so you always have something tasty to elevate basic ingredients.

Step 4: Use Meal "Templates" Instead of Recipes

One of the biggest planning mistakes is relying on new recipes every day. Instead, think in templates. A template is a basic meal format you can remix with different ingredients.

Try these hormone-friendly templates:

- Grain bowls: protein + veggies + grain + dressing
- Sheet-pan meals: protein + veggies + olive oil + seasoning, baked at 400°F
- Soups: broth + protein + veggies + herbs
- Wraps: collard leaves, nori, or tortillas + protein + veggie slaw + sauce
- Salad jars: greens + protein + seed topping + lemon vinaigrette

Rotate ingredients inside the templates instead of starting from scratch each week. This saves time, lowers stress, and keeps your plan flexible.

Step 5: Plan 2–3 Breakfasts and Lunches

You don't need a different breakfast every day. Choose 2 to 3 reliable options and rotate.

Examples:

- Chia pudding with berries and flax
- Eggs with spinach and avocado
- Protein smoothie with greens and nut butter
- Overnight oats with seeds and almond milk

Do the same for lunch. Choose bowls, salads, soups, or wraps that you enjoy and that hold up well if prepped in advance.

Step 6: Choose 4 Dinners and Leave Space

Trying to plan 7 unique dinners is often where the overwhelm begins. Instead, plan 4 hormone-supportive dinners. Leave the other nights open for:

- Leftovers
- Flex meals
- Dining out or ordering in with intention
- Breakfast-for-dinner options

Dinner ideas don't need to be fancy. You could rotate between:

- Sheet-pan salmon and Brussels sprouts
- Ground turkey lettuce wraps
- Coconut lentil stew
- Chicken over arugula with tahini dressing

> Planning fewer meals means
> less shopping,
> less waste,
> and more flexibility.

Step 7: Use Planning to Reduce Stress, Not Add It

If meal planning feels like pressure, scale it back. Some weeks, your plan might just be a protein + veggie combo for lunches and a few go-to dinners. Other weeks, you may prep more because life is full.

Use meal planning as a support system, not a rigid checklist. Your goal is not to follow a perfect plan but to avoid getting stuck in the "what's for dinner" panic that often leads to quick fixes that leave you inflamed or undernourished.

Sample 3-Day Plan Using This Method

Day 1

- Breakfast: Scrambled eggs with sautéed spinach and avocado
- Lunch: Leftover salmon grain bowl with arugula and tahini

- Dinner: Chicken sheet-pan with broccoli and carrots

Day 2

- Breakfast: Chia pudding with almond milk and berries
- Lunch: Lentil soup with side salad
- Dinner: Coconut curry with tofu and roasted cauliflower

Day 3

- Breakfast: Smoothie with protein, flax, and frozen berries
- Lunch: Turkey lettuce wraps with spicy slaw
- Dinner: Leftovers or breakfast-for-dinner with eggs and roasted sweet potatoes

3: Grocery List Strategy That Saves Time and Money

A good grocery list does more than organize your shopping. It removes decision fatigue, prevents waste, saves money, and makes hormone-supportive eating easier to follow through on. When your kitchen is stocked with the right ingredients, you're far more likely to make meals that heal instead of meals that derail.

You don't need a long list of specialty health foods to eat well. You need a clear plan, staple ingredients, and a way to shop with purpose. This section will walk you through how to build a smarter list, shop more efficiently, and support your goals without overspending or overbuying.

Start with a Master List by Section

One of the simplest ways to make grocery shopping faster and more focused is to organize your list by store layout or food category. Here's a basic template you can personalize:

Produce:

- Leafy greens (kale, arugula, spinach)
- Cruciferous veggies (broccoli, cauliflower, cabbage)
- Bell peppers, carrots, zucchini
- Sweet potatoes or winter squash
- Garlic, onions, leeks
- Berries, apples, citrus fruits

Protein:

- Eggs
- Chicken or turkey breast
- Wild-caught fish (fresh or frozen)

- Canned tuna or salmon
- Tofu or tempeh
- Lentils, black beans, chickpeas

Pantry Staples:

- Quinoa, brown rice, oats
- Chia seeds, flaxseed, pumpkin seeds
- Olive oil, coconut oil, tahini
- Apple cider vinegar, coconut aminos
- Low-sodium broth
- Canned tomatoes or beans

Dairy/Alternatives:

- Unsweetened almond or coconut milk
- Plain Greek yogurt or kefir
- Goat cheese or feta (optional)

Frozen:

- Frozen spinach, cauliflower, broccoli
- Berries and mango chunks
- Cooked grains or legume mixes
- Pre-cooked wild salmon fillets

Extras:

- Fresh herbs (cilantro, parsley, basil)
- Lemons and limes
- Herbal teas
- Natural sweeteners (stevia, monk fruit, or raw honey)

Use this template each week and add or subtract items based on what meals you're making and what you already have at home.

Shop Your Fridge and Pantry First

Before you create your grocery list, take 5 minutes to review what's already in your kitchen. This prevents you from buying duplicates, helps you use what's fresh, and inspires meals based on ingredients you already have.

Look for:

- Leftover proteins
- Veggies that need to be used
- Frozen items that can replace fresh
- Open containers or sauces to incorporate into meals

This quick habit not only saves money but helps reduce food waste, something that also supports your long-term sustainability mindset.

Plan to Shop Once a Week

Shopping once a week is ideal for most people. It saves time, allows you to batch prep effectively, and creates a predictable rhythm around meals. If needed, add a quick midweek refill trip for fresh greens or fruit, but let your main haul cover most of the week's meals.

Best shopping rhythm:

- Plan meals or outline your "template" for the week (see Section 2)
- Create your list based on your core proteins, veggies, and staples
- Shop once, prep once, and enjoy simpler cooking all week

Build In Flexibility: Plan for Substitutes

Always have a few flexible, multi-purpose items on your list that can fill in when something is out of stock or when a recipe changes. Good examples:

- Canned salmon if fresh fish is unavailable
- Frozen spinach in place of fresh
- Quinoa instead of brown rice
- Lentils as a backup protein

These flexible foods are also great to keep on hand for quick, no-plan meals when your week doesn't go as expected.

Budget Tips for Hormone-Friendly Eating

You don't need to break the bank to eat well. Here are strategies to keep your grocery bills aligned with your healing goals:

- Buy frozen vegetables and fruits: They're nutrient-dense, long-lasting, and often cheaper
- Buy in bulk: Stock up on dry goods like oats, rice, beans, and seeds when on sale
- Prioritize protein and produce: These two categories offer the biggest return for hormone health
- Shop store brands or local co-ops: Often more affordable than name-brand health foods

- Stretch ingredients: Use cooked chicken in multiple meals, or repurpose roasted veggies in salads, bowls, and wraps
- Avoid "health food hype": You don't need trendy powders or packaged superfoods to eat well. Real food is enough

Sample One-Week Grocery List

This example supports 4 dinners, 2 breakfasts, 2 lunch options, and snacks:

Produce:

- 2 bunches kale
- 1 bag arugula
- 2 sweet potatoes
- 1 head cauliflower
- 1 red bell pepper
- 1 zucchini
- 1 cucumber
- 1 red onion
- 2 garlic heads
- 2 lemons
- 1 avocado
- 1 pint blueberries
- 3 apples

Protein:

- 1 dozen pasture-raised eggs
- 1 lb chicken breast
- 1 lb ground turkey
- 2 cans wild salmon
- 1 block tofu
- 1 cup dry lentils

Pantry & Other:

- Olive oil
- Quinoa
- Steel-cut oats

- Chia seeds
- Almond butter
- Tahini
- Coconut milk
- Apple cider vinegar
- Sea salt and spices (turmeric, paprika, cumin)

Frozen:

- 1 bag frozen broccoli
- 1 bag frozen spinach
- 1 bag frozen blueberries

This list supports a variety of meals with minimal prep and maximum flexibility.

4: Batch Cooking and Meal Prep Shortcuts

Meal prep isn't just for bodybuilders and food bloggers. For women over 40 trying to balance hormones, reduce inflammation, and stay energized, it's one of the most powerful tools for staying consistent, without having to cook from scratch every night.

The goal is not to prep every meal for the week. It's to create building blocks you can mix and match into quick, satisfying meals when life gets busy.

Let's walk through how to batch cook and prep like a pro, without spending your whole weekend in the kitchen.

The "Cook Once, Eat Often" Strategy

Think of batch cooking as meal foundations. When you prepare core components in advance, assembling meals during the week takes just minutes.

The basics include:

- 2–3 proteins
- 2–3 roasted or steamed veggies
- 1 or 2 complex carbs
- 1 to 2 sauces or dressings
- A few grab-and-go extras (hard-boiled eggs, chia pudding, smoothie packs)

From there, you can build dozens of combinations: bowls, wraps, salads, soups, and one-pan dinners.

Batch Proteins to Build Your Meals

Choose 2 or 3 proteins each week and prep them in a way that makes them easy to reheat or repurpose.

Examples:

- Roast a tray of salmon fillets with lemon and dill
- Grill or bake chicken breast with olive oil and spices
- Sauté ground turkey with garlic and greens
- Cook a big batch of lentils or chickpeas for bowls and soups
- Boil a half dozen eggs for snacks and breakfasts

Store cooked proteins in glass containers in the fridge. Most will last 3 to 4 days. Freeze extra portions to extend their shelf life.

Prep Veggie Bases in Bulk

Cooked vegetables are easy to reheat, add to meals, or eat cold in salads.

Simple veggie prep ideas:

- Roast broccoli, cauliflower, and carrots with olive oil and turmeric
- Steam a batch of kale or spinach for easy sides or omelets
- Bake cubed sweet potato with cinnamon and sea salt
- Chop a container of raw peppers, cucumbers, and cherry tomatoes for quick salads or snacks

Line your sheet pans, season once, and roast multiple veggies at the same time to save time and effort.

Cook Your Grains or Starches in Advance

Having a grain or complex carb ready gives you instant meal power. Make one or two to use in different ways:

- Cook quinoa and store in glass jars for salads and bowls
- Make a batch of steel-cut oats for the next few breakfasts
- Bake extra sweet potatoes to reheat with lunch or dinner
- Cook brown rice or wild rice for stir-fries, soups, or sides

Stick to unprocessed, fiber-rich starches to keep blood sugar stable.

Make One or Two Sauces to Elevate Everything

Healthy sauces and dressings turn basic ingredients into flavorful meals. Keep a few homemade or clean-store versions on hand.

Easy sauce ideas:

- Lemon tahini dressing
- Olive oil and balsamic vinaigrette
- Greek yogurt with garlic and dill
- Avocado-lime sauce
- Almond butter coconut sauce for grain bowls

Store in small jars and use within 5 days. A good sauce makes leftovers feel fresh again.

Store and Label for Ease

A few storage tips make all the difference:

- Use clear glass containers so you can see what you have
- Label items with masking tape or a marker (protein, date cooked)
- Store items by category (protein in one shelf section, veggies in another)
- Use small containers for pre-portioned snacks (seeds, nuts, fruit, hard-boiled eggs)

Having a neat, organized fridge removes friction and invites healthy decisions.

Sample 90-Minute Meal Prep Flow

If you have just 90 minutes to prep for the week, here's what you can do:

- Step 1 (0–10 mins): Preheat oven to 400°F, rinse grains and chop veggies
- Step 2 (10–30 mins): Start cooking grains (quinoa, rice, oats) on the stovetop
- Step 3 (30–60 mins): Place salmon, chicken, and veggies on sheet pans and bake
- Step 4 (60–75 mins): Hard-boil eggs, make chia pudding or smoothie packs

Step 5 (75–90 mins): Whisk together dressings or sauces and clean up

You'll walk away with proteins, grains, veggies, snacks, and sauces that can feed you for 4 to 5 days.

Make It Work for Your Life

Some weeks you'll prep more. Other weeks, you'll barely prep at all. That's normal. Instead of focusing on perfection, aim to prep just enough to support your body.

When you're short on time:

- Buy pre-cut veggies and salad kits
- Use rotisserie chicken (remove the skin and choose organic if possible)

- Keep frozen options on hand for emergency meals
- Use protein powders or bars for fast backup fuel

The goal is always nourishment, not performance.

5: What to Eat When Life Falls Apart

There will be weeks when nothing goes according to plan.

You'll skip the grocery store. You'll forget what's in the fridge. You'll feel too tired to cook, too overwhelmed to care, or too stressed to think clearly about what your body actually needs.

This doesn't mean you've failed. It means you're human. And if your nutrition plan can't handle your messiest weeks, it's not sustainable.

The Galveston approach is built to create enough structure and compassion to return to nourishment, no matter how far you drift.

Here's how to feed yourself when everything falls apart.

Build a Back-Up Nutrition Kit

The key to surviving chaotic weeks is having an "emergency stash" of nourishing foods that require little to no prep. These foods won't win culinary awards, but they will support your hormones, stabilize your energy, and prevent the blood sugar crashes that lead to overeating or emotional snacking.

Fridge-friendly backups:

- Hard-boiled eggs
- Washed greens
- Pre-cooked lentils or beans
- Greek yogurt or kefir
- Cooked quinoa or brown rice
- Leftover soup in mason jars

Freezer lifesavers:

- Frozen wild salmon or shrimp
- Frozen chopped veggies (broccoli, spinach, stir-fry blends)
- Pre-made smoothie packs
- Bone broth cubes
- Cooked chicken thighs or turkey meatballs

Pantry staples:

- Canned salmon or tuna
- Nut butters
- Chia seeds
- Rice cakes
- Low-sodium lentil or vegetable soup
- Herbal teas

These ingredients form the foundation of no-brainer meals when cooking feels impossible.

10-Minute Meal Ideas for Zero Bandwidth Days

Sometimes just the thought of making food is exhausting. Here are a few go-to options that require minimal thought and deliver maximum nourishment:

1. The "power plate":

- 2 boiled eggs or canned tuna
- A handful of greens with olive oil and lemon
- A slice of avocado or a spoonful of tahini
- Crackers or leftover rice for carbs

2. Smoothie meal:

- Unsweetened almond milk, protein powder, frozen berries, chia seeds
- Add nut butter or avocado for staying power

3. Soup and topper:

- Heat a lentil or veggie-based soup
- Add olive oil and pumpkin seeds
- Pair with a side of roasted sweet potato or salad

4. Fast bowl:

- Microwave frozen veggies
- Add pre-cooked grains and protein
- Top with dressing or coconut aminos

5. Breakfast for dinner:

- Scrambled eggs with spinach and salsa
- Side of berries or toast with ghee

These meals aren't glamorous. But they're nutrient-dense, grounding, and easy to repeat.

Eating Out or Ordering In Without Starting Over

Sometimes the best choice is ordering a meal. The goal is not to eat perfectly. It's to avoid meals that leave you inflamed, exhausted, or mentally foggy.

When dining out or ordering in:

- Choose grilled over fried
- Ask for sauces or dressings on the side
- Swap the starch for veggies or a side salad
- Avoid creamy or sugary drinks
- Eat until satisfied—not stuffed
- Balance indulgences with water, fiber, or extra veggies later that day

You can enjoy your meal and still honor your body. A single takeout meal is not failure but part of real life.

When You Fall Off Completely

There may be days when you reach for sugar, skip meals, drink too much coffee, and go to bed feeling like you lost all your progress.

This is not the end.

Your body isn't keeping score. It's listening. And it responds beautifully to your next choice. You don't need to compensate, punish, or start over. You just need to return to the habits that help you feel good.

- Ask:
- What's one grounding meal I can make today?
- What will help me feel more hydrated, calm, or supported?

What's the next doable thing, even if it's not the perfect one?

Healing isn't linear. But it is always available.

Your Life, Nourished by Design

You've just built something powerful: a system that supports your healing, even when life doesn't go as planned.

No more relying on willpower alone. No more getting caught in the "what should I eat?" spiral that drains your energy before you even open the fridge. Now, you have rhythms. You have anchors. You have meals and strategies that work with your hormones, not against them.

This chapter wasn't about getting everything prepped perfectly or following a rigid routine. It was about learning how to design a week that makes nourishment easy to choose. That gives you something to fall back on when things feel overwhelming. That removes the friction between your goals and your real life.

You don't need more rules. You need fewer decisions. You need meals that feel familiar, ingredients that are already in your kitchen, and a plan that honors your energy.

And now, you have it.

CHAPTER 9: RECIPES FOR HORMONE RESET, FAT BURNING & ENERGY BOOST

I. Energizing Breakfasts

Supports: Fat loss, hormone balance, metabolism reset, and morning energy boost

1. Mary Claire's Parfait or Smoothie

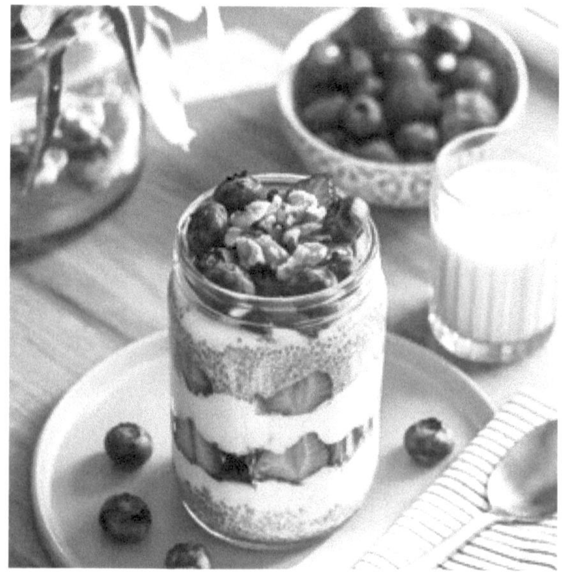

MAKES 1 SERVING

INGREDIENTS:

- 1 cup plain Greek yogurt (full-fat)
- 2 tablespoons fresh blueberries
- 2 tablespoons fresh strawberries, sliced
- 1 tablespoon chia seeds
- 1 tablespoon chopped walnuts
- 1 teaspoon honey (optional)
- ½ cup unsweetened almond milk (for smoothie)

1 teaspoon vanilla extract (for smoothie)

INSTRUCTIONS:

1. For Parfait: In a tall glass or jar, layer half the Greek yogurt, followed by half the blueberries, strawberries, chia seeds, and walnuts. Repeat the layers.
2. Drizzle with honey if desired.
3. Serve immediately or chill for 10 minutes to let flavors meld.
4. For Smoothie: Combine Greek yogurt, blueberries, strawberries, chia seeds, walnuts, almond milk, and vanilla extract in a blender.
5. Blend on high for 30–45 seconds until smooth. If too thick, add more almond milk, 1 tablespoon at a time, until desired consistency is reached.
6. Pour into a glass and serve immediately, or store in a sealed container for up to 24 hours.

2. Egg Scramble

MAKES 1 SERVING

INGREDIENTS:

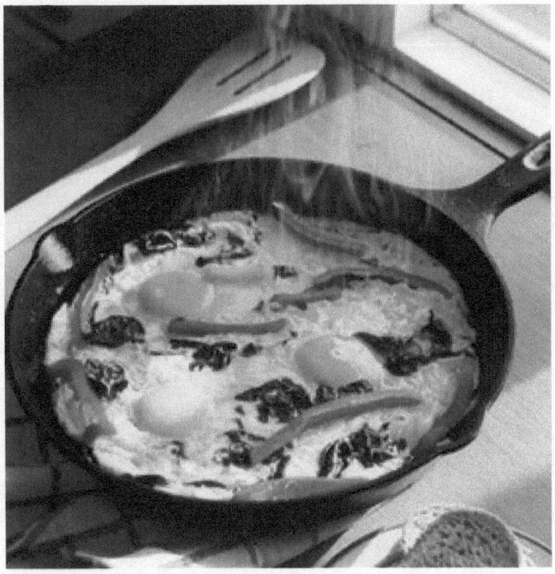

- 2 large eggs
- 1 tablespoon olive oil
- ¼ cup diced bell peppers (red or yellow)
- ¼ cup chopped spinach
- 2 tablespoons diced onion
- 1 tablespoon shredded cheddar cheese
- Salt and black pepper to taste

1 teaspoon fresh parsley, chopped (optional)

INSTRUCTIONS:

1. Heat olive oil in a nonstick skillet over medium heat.
2. Add bell peppers and onion; sauté for 3–4 minutes until softened.
3. Add spinach and cook for 1 minute until wilted.
4. In a bowl, whisk eggs with salt and pepper.
5. Pour into skillet and stir gently. Cook for 2–3 minutes until just set.
6. Sprinkle in cheddar cheese; stir until melted.
7. Remove from heat and garnish with parsley if desired.
8. Serve immediately with a side of toast or fruit.

3. Cottage Cheese Omelet

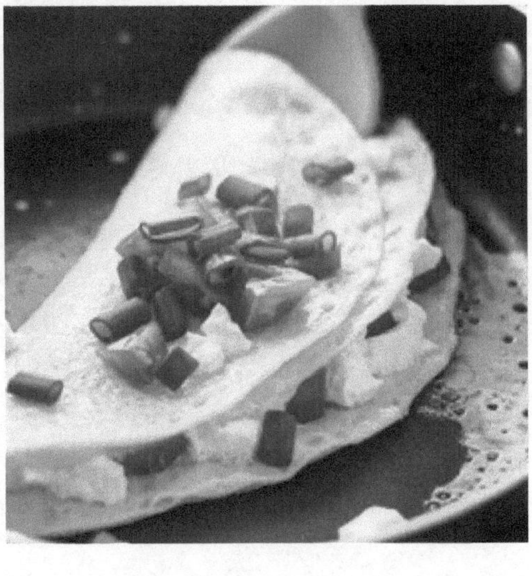

MAKES 1 SERVING

INGREDIENTS:

- 2 large eggs
- ¼ cup cottage cheese (full-fat)
- 1 tablespoon butter
- 2 tablespoons diced tomatoes
- 1 tablespoon chopped green onions
- Salt and black pepper to taste

½ teaspoon dried dill (optional)

INSTRUCTIONS:

1. In a bowl, whisk eggs with salt, pepper, and dill until well combined.
2. Heat butter in a nonstick skillet over medium-low heat.
3. Pour in eggs, swirling to coat the pan evenly.
4. Cook for 2–3 minutes until edges begin to set.
5. Spoon cottage cheese, tomatoes, and green onions over one half.
6. Fold the other half of the omelet over the filling.
7. Cook another 1–2 minutes until fully set but not overcooked.
8. Slide onto a plate and serve with salad or avocado.

4. Poached Eggs with Cabbage Hash Browns

MAKES 1 SERVING

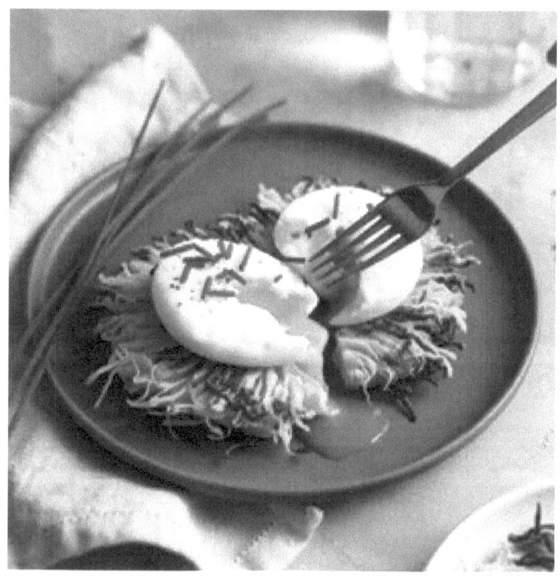

INGREDIENTS:

- 2 large eggs
- 2 cups shredded cabbage
- 2 tablespoons olive oil
- ¼ cup diced onion
- 1 teaspoon garlic powder
- Salt and black pepper to taste
- 1 tablespoon white vinegar

1 teaspoon fresh chives, chopped (optional)

INSTRUCTIONS:

1. For Hash Browns: Heat olive oil in a skillet over medium heat.
2. Add cabbage, onion, garlic powder, salt, and pepper.
3. Cook 8–10 minutes, stirring occasionally, until golden and crispy.
4. Set aside.
5. For Poached Eggs: Fill a saucepan with water, add vinegar, and bring to a gentle simmer.
6. Crack eggs into small bowls.
7. Stir water to create a whirlpool, slide eggs in.

8. Cook 3–4 minutes until whites are set but yolks are runny.
9. Remove with a slotted spoon and drain.
10. Serve eggs over cabbage hash browns. Garnish with chives if using.

5. Avocado "For Life" Toast

MAKES 1 SERVING

INGREDIENTS:

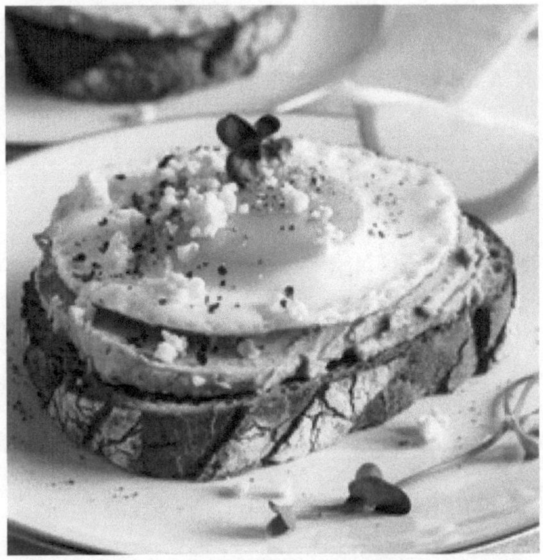

- 1 slice whole-grain or low-carb bread
- ½ ripe avocado
- 1 large egg
- 1 tablespoon olive oil
- 1 tablespoon crumbled feta cheese
- 1 teaspoon lemon juice
- Pinch of red pepper flakes (optional)

Salt and black pepper to taste

INSTRUCTIONS:

1. Toast the bread until golden and crisp.
2. In a small bowl, mash avocado with lemon juice, salt, and pepper.
3. Spread avocado mixture over the toast.
4. Heat olive oil in a skillet over medium heat.
5. Fry the egg to desired doneness (about 2–3 minutes).
6. Place the egg on top of the avocado toast.
7. Sprinkle with feta and red pepper flakes if using.
8. Serve with fresh greens or cherry tomatoes.

This toast is rich in healthy fats from avocado, protein from the egg, and tangy flavor from feta, making it a deliciously balanced start to the day.

6. Flaxseed Pancakes

MAKES 1 SERVING

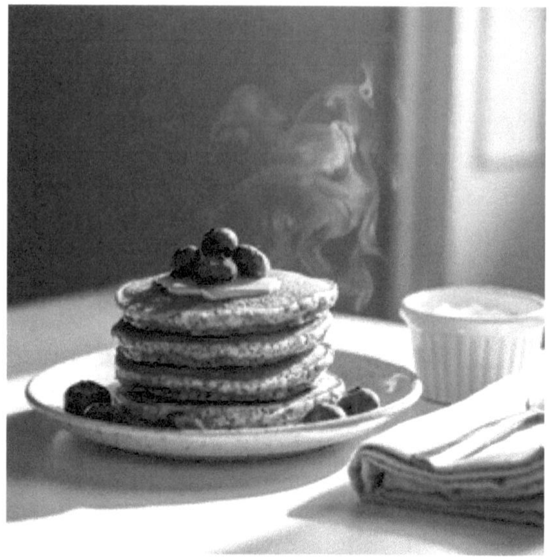

INGREDIENTS:

- 2 large eggs
- ¼ cup ground flaxseed
- 2 tablespoons unsweetened almond milk
- 1 tablespoon coconut oil, melted
- ½ teaspoon baking powder
- ¼ teaspoon ground cinnamon
- 1 teaspoon monk fruit sweetener

1 tablespoon blueberries (optional topping)

INSTRUCTIONS:

1. In a bowl, whisk together eggs, almond milk, and melted coconut oil.
2. Add flaxseed, baking powder, cinnamon, and monk fruit sweetener. Stir until thick batter forms.
3. Heat a nonstick skillet over medium heat and lightly grease with coconut oil.
4. Pour batter to form two small pancakes.
5. Cook each side for 2–3 minutes until golden and set.
6. Serve warm, topped with blueberries if desired.
7. Optionally pair with full-fat Greek yogurt for added protein.

These grain-free pancakes are rich in omega-3s and healthy fats, making them a fiber-packed and satisfying low-carb breakfast aligned with the Galveston Diet.

7. Pumpkin Pancakes

MAKES 1 SERVING

INGREDIENTS:

- ¼ cup pumpkin puree
- 2 large eggs
- 2 tablespoons almond flour
- 1 tablespoon ground flaxseed
- ½ teaspoon baking powder
- ¼ teaspoon ground nutmeg

- ½ teaspoon monk fruit sweetener
- 1 tablespoon coconut oil

1 tablespoon chopped pecans (optional topping)

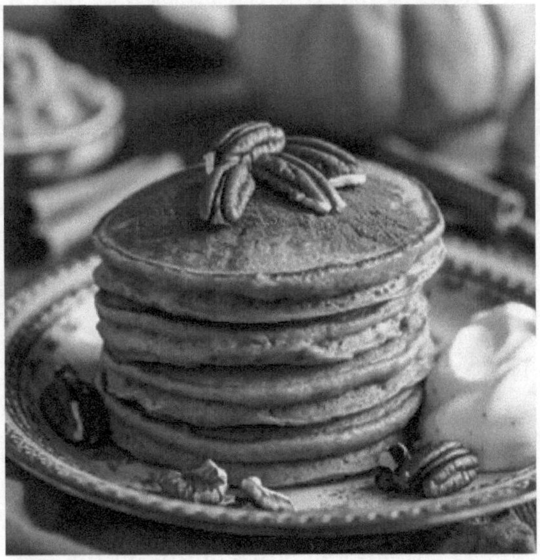

INSTRUCTIONS:

1. In a bowl, whisk together pumpkin puree, eggs, almond flour, flaxseed, baking powder, nutmeg, and monk fruit.
2. Heat coconut oil in a nonstick skillet over medium heat.
3. Pour batter into the skillet to form two pancakes.
4. Cook 3–4 minutes per side until firm and browned.
5. Top with pecans if desired.
6. Pair with unsweetened coconut yogurt for creaminess.

These pancakes offer fiber from pumpkin, a grain-free base from almond flour, and sweet warmth from nutmeg. They're low-carb and anti-inflammatory.

8. Breakfast Salad

MAKES 1 SERVING

INGREDIENTS:

- 2 cups baby spinach
- 1 large egg, hard-boiled
- ¼ avocado, sliced
- 2 tablespoons cherry tomatoes, halved
- 1 tablespoon sliced almonds
- 1 tablespoon olive oil
- 1 teaspoon lemon juice
- ¼ teaspoon ground turmeric

Salt and black pepper to taste

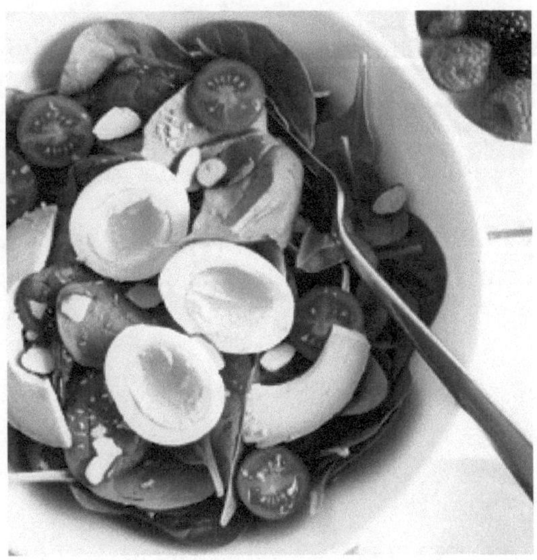

INSTRUCTIONS:

1. Place spinach in a bowl.
2. Slice the hard-boiled egg and add on top along with avocado and tomatoes.
3. Sprinkle with sliced almonds.

4. In a small bowl, whisk olive oil, lemon juice, turmeric, salt, and pepper.
5. Drizzle dressing over the salad and toss gently.
6. Serve immediately. Optionally pair with berries on the side.

This salad is rich in greens, protein, and healthy fats, with anti-inflammatory turmeric for added benefit. A colorful, satisfying start to your day.

9. Blueberry Pie Smoothie

MAKES 1 SERVING

INGREDIENTS:

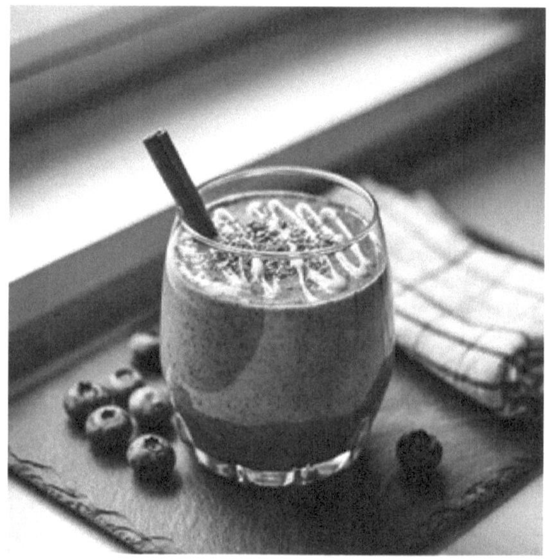

- ½ cup fresh blueberries
- ½ cup unsweetened almond milk
- ¼ cup full-fat Greek yogurt
- 1 tablespoon ground flaxseed
- 1 tablespoon almond butter
- ¼ teaspoon ground cinnamon
- ½ teaspoon monk fruit sweetener

2 ice cubes

INSTRUCTIONS:

1. Add all ingredients to a blender.
2. Blend on high for 30–45 seconds until smooth and creamy.
3. If too thick, add more almond milk 1 tablespoon at a time.
4. Pour into a glass and serve immediately, or refrigerate for up to 24 hours.

This smoothie is packed with low-sugar fruit, protein, and healthy fats. It's quick, energizing, and anti-inflammatory—perfect for breakfast or post-workout.

10. Mixed Berry Smoothie

MAKES 1 SERVING

INGREDIENTS:

- ¼ cup fresh strawberries
- ¼ cup fresh raspberries
- ¼ cup fresh blueberries

- ½ cup unsweetened coconut milk
- 1 tablespoon chia seeds
- 1 tablespoon collagen powder (optional)
- ½ teaspoon vanilla extract
- ½ teaspoon monk fruit sweetener

2 ice cubes

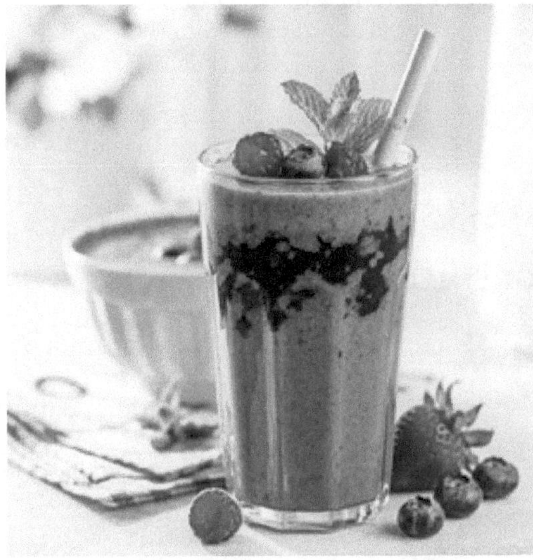

INSTRUCTIONS:

1. Add berries, coconut milk, chia seeds, collagen (if using), vanilla, monk fruit, and ice to a blender.
2. Blend on high for 30–45 seconds until smooth.
3. Adjust thickness with more coconut milk as needed.
4. Pour into a glass and serve immediately, or refrigerate for later.

This triple-berry smoothie is rich in antioxidants, fiber, and healthy fats, supporting inflammation control and sustained energy throughout your morning.

11. Raspberry Almond Smoothie

MAKES 1 SERVING

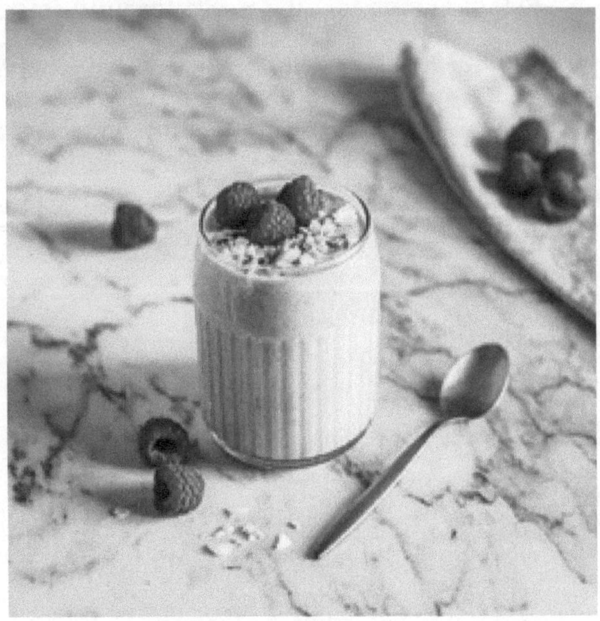

INGREDIENTS:

- ½ cup fresh raspberries
- ½ cup unsweetened almond milk
- 1 tablespoon almond butter
- ¼ cup full-fat Greek yogurt
- 1 tablespoon ground flaxseed
- ½ teaspoon vanilla extract
- ½ teaspoon monk fruit sweetener

2 ice cubes

INSTRUCTIONS:

1. Add raspberries, almond milk, almond butter, Greek yogurt, flaxseed, vanilla, monk fruit, and ice cubes to a blender.
2. Blend on high for 30–45 seconds until smooth and creamy.
3. If too thick, add almond milk 1 tablespoon at a time to adjust consistency.
4. Pour into a glass and serve immediately, or store in a sealed container for up to 24 hours.

This smoothie is quick, satisfying, and anti-inflammatory, featuring healthy fats, fiber, and protein with a sweet berry flavor and no added sugar.

12. Peanut Butter Cup Smoothie

MAKES 1 SERVING

INGREDIENTS:

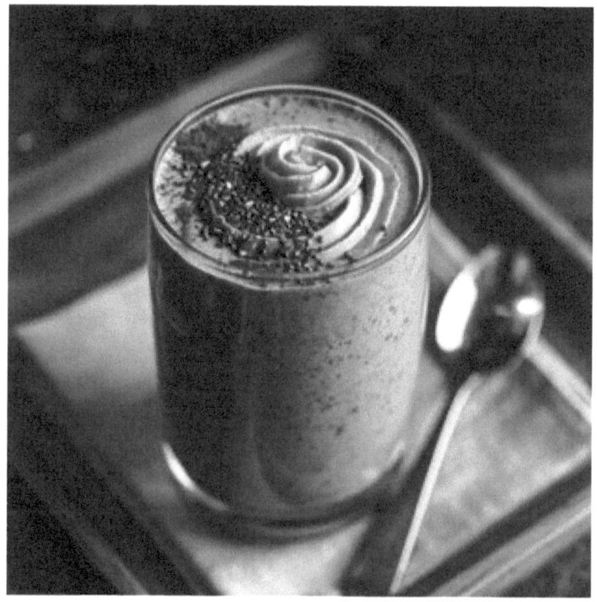

- ½ cup unsweetened coconut milk
- 1 tablespoon no-sugar-added peanut butter
- 1 tablespoon unsweetened cocoa powder
- ¼ cup full-fat Greek yogurt
- 1 tablespoon chia seeds
- ½ teaspoon monk fruit sweetener
- ¼ teaspoon vanilla extract

2 ice cubes

INSTRUCTIONS:

1. Combine all ingredients in a blender.
2. Blend on high for 30–45 seconds until smooth.
3. Add more coconut milk as needed to reach desired thickness.
4. Pour into a glass and enjoy immediately or refrigerate for later.

This creamy, chocolatey smoothie satisfies sweet cravings while fueling your body with protein, fiber, and healthy fats. It's a nutrient-dense, sugar-free breakfast.

13. Peanut Butter–Mocha Smoothie

MAKES 1 SERVING

INGREDIENTS:

- ½ cup unsweetened almond milk
- ¼ cup brewed coffee, cooled
- 1 tablespoon no-sugar-added peanut butter
- 1 tablespoon unsweetened cocoa powder
- 1 tablespoon ground flaxseed
- ½ teaspoon monk fruit sweetener

- ¼ teaspoon vanilla extract

2 ice cubes

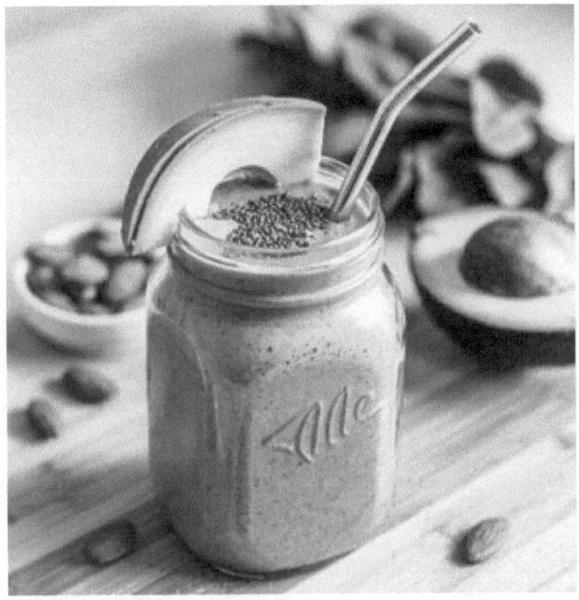

INSTRUCTIONS:

1. Add almond milk, coffee, peanut butter, cocoa, flaxseed, monk fruit, vanilla, and ice to a blender.
2. Blend on high until smooth and frothy.
3. Adjust with additional almond milk if needed for consistency.
4. Pour into a glass and serve immediately or store in the fridge for up to 24 hours.

This energizing smoothie blends caffeine, protein, and healthy fats to keep you full and focused without sugar crashes.

14. Green Almond Butter Smoothie

MAKES 1 SERVING

INGREDIENTS:

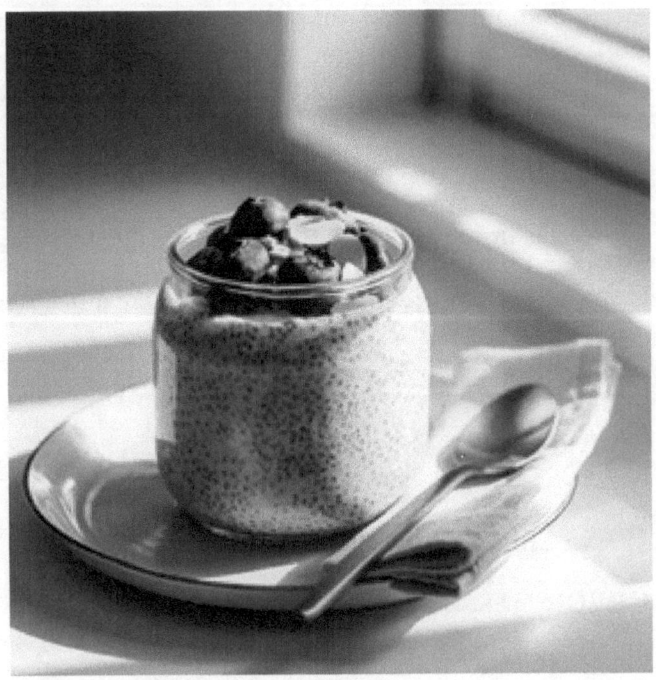

- ½ cup unsweetened coconut milk
- 1 cup baby spinach
- 1 tablespoon almond butter
- ¼ avocado
- 1 tablespoon chia seeds
- ½ teaspoon monk fruit sweetener
- ¼ teaspoon ground cinnamon

2 ice cubes

INSTRUCTIONS:

1. Add coconut milk, spinach, almond butter, avocado, chia seeds, monk fruit, cinnamon, and ice to a blender.
2. Blend on high for 30–45 seconds until smooth.
3. Add more coconut milk 1 tablespoon at a time if too thick.
4. Pour into a glass and serve immediately or chill in a sealed container.

This green smoothie is rich in antioxidants, fiber, and healthy fats, making it an ideal anti-inflammatory start to your morning.

15. Vegan Cinnamon Roll Smoothie

MAKES 1 SERVING

INGREDIENTS:

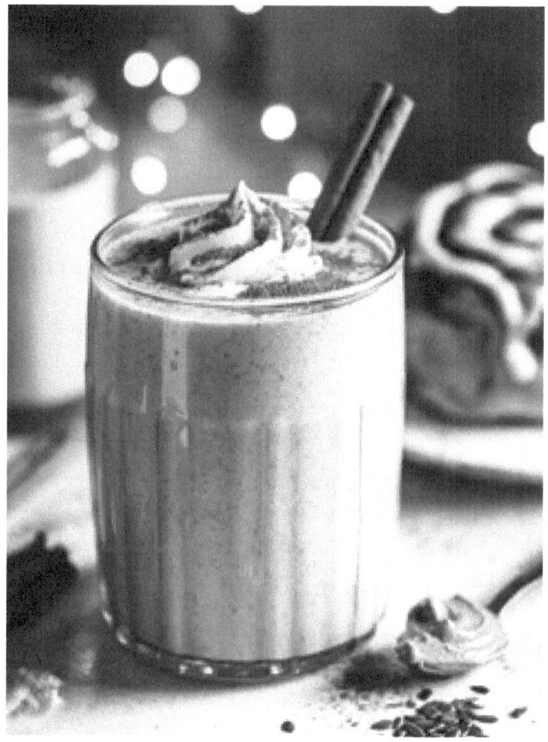

- ½ cup unsweetened almond milk
- 1 tablespoon almond butter
- 1 tablespoon ground flaxseed
- ½ frozen banana (small)
- ½ teaspoon ground cinnamon
- ½ teaspoon vanilla extract
- ½ teaspoon monk fruit sweetener

2 ice cubes

INSTRUCTIONS:

1. Combine almond milk, almond butter, flaxseed, banana, cinnamon, vanilla, monk fruit, and ice in a blender.
2. Blend on high until creamy and smooth.
3. Adjust thickness with extra almond milk if desired.
4. Serve immediately or store in the fridge for up to 24 hours.

This smoothie tastes like dessert but fuels like a balanced meal, packed with healthy fats, fiber, and flavor, without the sugar.

16. Chia Pudding

MAKES 1 SERVING

INGREDIENTS:

- 2 tablespoons chia seeds
- ½ cup unsweetened almond milk
- ½ teaspoon vanilla extract
- ½ teaspoon monk fruit sweetener
- 1 tablespoon sliced almonds

1 tablespoon fresh blueberries

INSTRUCTIONS:

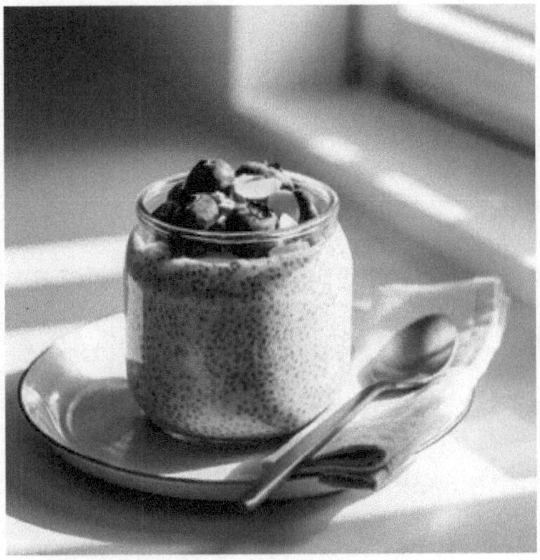

1. In a small bowl or jar, combine chia seeds, almond milk, vanilla extract, and monk fruit sweetener.
2. Stir well to prevent clumping.
3. Cover and refrigerate for at least 4 hours or overnight. Stir once halfway through.
4. Before serving, top with sliced almonds and blueberries.
5. Serve chilled as a standalone breakfast or with a side of hard-boiled eggs.

This Galveston Diet-friendly breakfast is rich in fiber, omega-3s, and healthy fats. It's light, filling, and easy to prep ahead.

17. Coconut–Chia Pudding with Raspberries

MAKES 1 SERVING

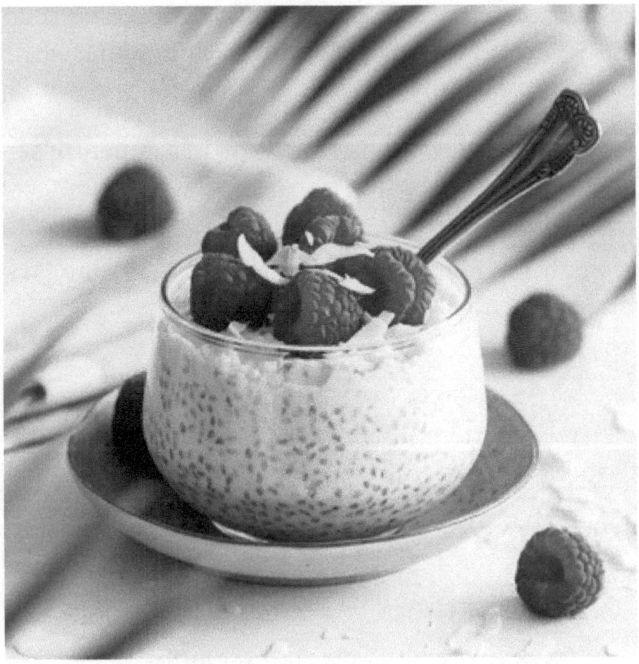

INGREDIENTS:

- 2 tablespoons chia seeds
- ½ cup unsweetened coconut milk
- ½ teaspoon vanilla extract
- ½ teaspoon monk fruit sweetener
- ¼ cup fresh raspberries

1 tablespoon unsweetened coconut flakes

INSTRUCTIONS:

1. In a bowl or jar, mix chia seeds, coconut milk, vanilla extract, and monk fruit sweetener.
2. Stir thoroughly to avoid clumps.
3. Cover and refrigerate for 4 hours or overnight, stirring once halfway.
4. Top with raspberries and coconut flakes before serving.
5. Serve chilled, optionally with a handful of walnuts for added fat.

This creamy, low-sugar pudding is perfect for hormone support and blood sugar stability with fiber, healthy fat, and antioxidants.

18. Coconut and Walnut Chia Pudding

MAKES 1 SERVING

INGREDIENTS:

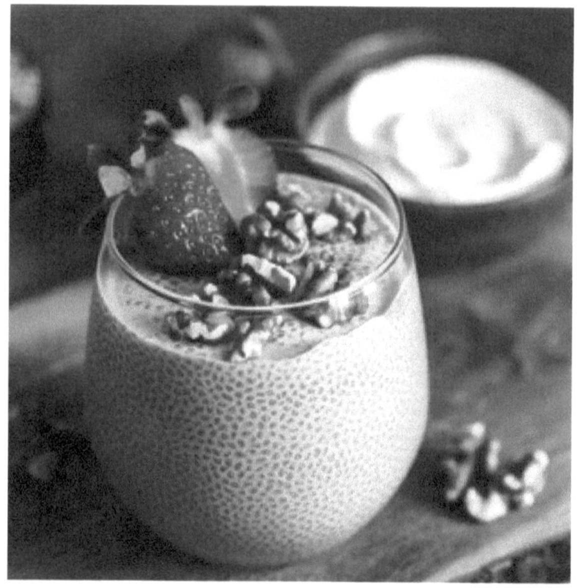

- 2 tablespoons chia seeds
- ½ cup unsweetened coconut milk
- ½ teaspoon monk fruit sweetener
- ¼ teaspoon ground cinnamon
- 1 tablespoon chopped walnuts

1 tablespoon fresh strawberries, sliced

INSTRUCTIONS:

1. In a bowl or jar, mix chia seeds, coconut milk, monk fruit, and cinnamon.
2. Stir well to combine.
3. Cover and refrigerate for 4+ hours or overnight, stirring once during chilling.
4. Top with walnuts and strawberries before serving.
5. Optionally, pair with full-fat Greek yogurt for extra protein.

This high-fat, high-fiber breakfast is both creamy and satisfying, with warm spice and subtle sweetness.

19. Peanut Butter and Chocolate Chia Pudding

MAKES 1 SERVING

INGREDIENTS:

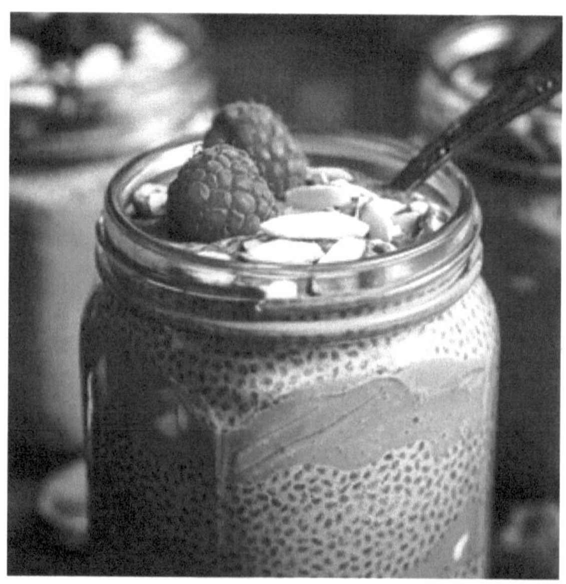

- 2 tablespoons chia seeds
- ½ cup unsweetened almond milk
- 1 tablespoon no-sugar-added peanut butter
- 1 teaspoon unsweetened cocoa powder
- ½ teaspoon monk fruit sweetener
- ½ teaspoon vanilla extract

1 tablespoon sliced almonds

INSTRUCTIONS:

1. Combine chia seeds, almond milk, peanut butter, cocoa powder, monk fruit, and vanilla in a jar or

bowl.

2. Stir thoroughly until well blended.

3. Cover and refrigerate for 4 hours or overnight, stirring once during chilling.

4. Top with sliced almonds before serving.

5. Optionally, serve with a few raspberries.

This indulgent-tasting recipe is loaded with healthy fats and fiber and keeps you full without added sugar.

20. Chocolate Peanut Butter Yogurt

MAKES 1 SERVING

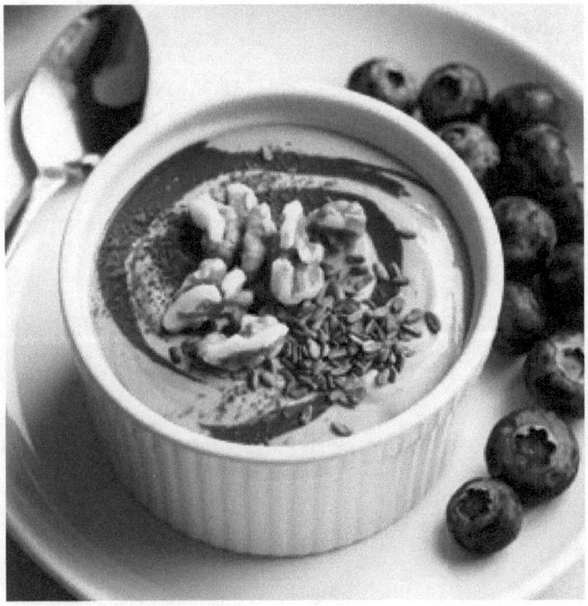

INGREDIENTS:

- ½ cup full-fat Greek yogurt
- 1 tablespoon no-sugar-added peanut butter
- 1 teaspoon unsweetened cocoa powder
- ½ teaspoon monk fruit sweetener
- 1 tablespoon ground flaxseed

1 tablespoon chopped walnuts

INSTRUCTIONS:

1. In a small bowl, combine Greek yogurt, peanut butter, cocoa powder, and monk fruit sweetener. Mix until smooth.

2. Stir in flaxseed.

3. Top with chopped walnuts.

4. Serve immediately or chill for 10 minutes.

5. Optionally pair with a few blueberries for antioxidants.

A rich and creamy high-protein breakfast that's both satisfying and anti-inflammatory—perfect for busy mornings.

21. Vegan Yogurt Parfait

MAKES 1 SERVING

INGREDIENTS:

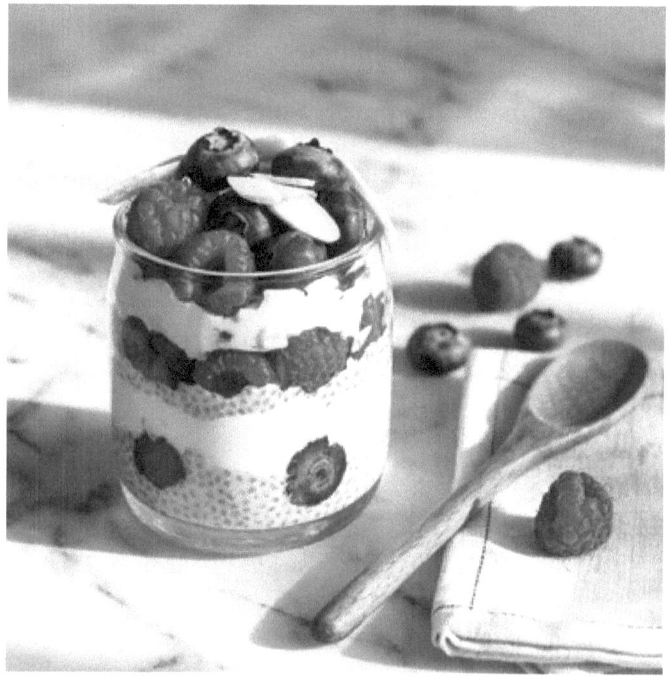

- ½ cup unsweetened coconut yogurt
- ¼ cup fresh raspberries
- 2 tablespoons fresh blueberries
- 1 tablespoon chia seeds
- 1 tablespoon sliced almonds

½ teaspoon monk fruit sweetener

INSTRUCTIONS:

1. In a small glass or jar, layer half the coconut yogurt, followed by half the raspberries, blueberries, chia seeds, and almonds.
2. Repeat the layers with the remaining ingredients.
3. Sprinkle monk fruit sweetener on top.
4. Serve immediately or chill for 10–15 minutes to let flavors meld.
5. Optional: Pair with a handful of walnuts for added healthy fats.

This dairy-free, high-fat parfait is rich in fiber and antioxidants, making it a quick, anti-inflammatory breakfast that's creamy and satisfying.

22. Raspberry-Flax Muffin

MAKES 1 SERVING

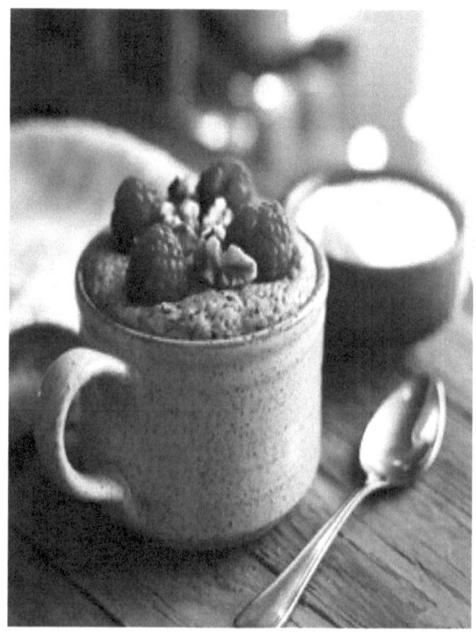

INGREDIENTS:

- 1 large egg
- 1 tablespoon coconut oil, melted
- 1 teaspoon vanilla extract
- 4 tablespoons ground flaxseed
- ½ teaspoon baking powder
- ¼ teaspoon ground cinnamon
- ½ teaspoon monk fruit sweetener
- 2 tablespoons fresh raspberries

1 tablespoon chopped walnuts

INSTRUCTIONS:

1. In a microwave-safe mug, whisk egg, coconut oil, and vanilla extract.
2. Add flaxseed, baking powder, cinnamon, and monk fruit sweetener. Stir until smooth.
3. Gently fold in raspberries and walnuts.
4. Microwave on high for 90 seconds, or until set.
5. Let cool slightly before eating. Optionally, serve with unsweetened coconut yogurt.

This grain-free muffin is rich in omega-3s, healthy fats, and fiber. It's a warm, quick-fix breakfast that satisfies and supports hormone health.

II. Midday Power Lunches

Supports: Blood sugar control, stress management, sustained energy, and anti-inflammatory eating

23. Chicken and BLT Wrap

MAKES 1 SERVING

INGREDIENTS:

- 1 large lettuce leaf (e.g., romaine or butter lettuce)
- 3 oz grilled chicken breast, sliced
- 2 slices nitrate-free bacon, cooked
- ¼ cup cherry tomatoes, halved
- ¼ avocado, sliced
- 1 tablespoon olive oil mayonnaise
- 1 teaspoon chopped fresh basil

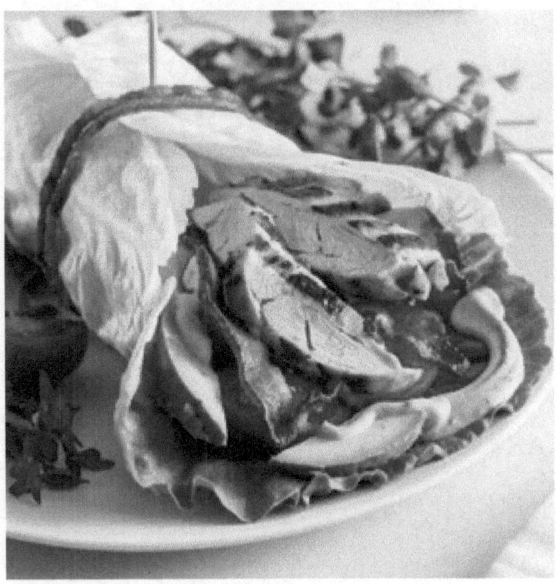

INSTRUCTIONS:

1. Lay the lettuce leaf flat on a plate.
2. Spread olive oil mayo over the center.
3. Add grilled chicken, bacon, cherry tomatoes, and avocado slices.
4. Sprinkle with fresh basil.
5. Roll the lettuce around the filling to form a wrap.
6. Secure with a toothpick and serve.

This low-carb wrap is packed with protein and healthy fats while skipping refined carbs, a perfect portable Galveston-friendly meal.

24. Tuna Salad with Snacky Side Salad

MAKES 1 SERVING

INGREDIENTS:

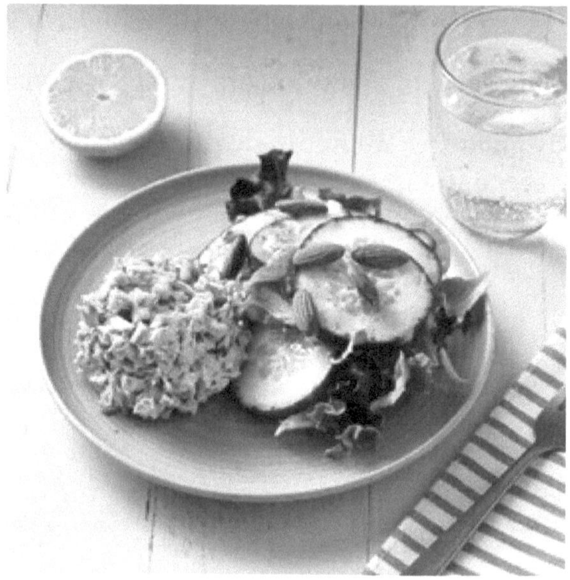

- 1 can (5 oz) tuna in water, drained
- 1 tablespoon olive oil mayonnaise
- 1 teaspoon Dijon mustard
- ¼ cup diced celery
- 2 cups mixed greens
- ¼ cup cucumber, sliced
- 1 tablespoon olive oil
- 1 teaspoon lemon juice

Salt and black pepper to taste

INSTRUCTIONS:

1. In a small bowl, combine tuna, mayo, mustard, and celery. Mix well and season with salt and pepper.
2. In a separate bowl, toss greens and cucumber with olive oil and lemon juice.
3. Serve tuna over greens or alongside.
4. Optional: Add sliced almonds for extra crunch.

This balanced lunch delivers protein, fiber, and healthy fats without the carbs—quick to prep and refreshing to eat.

25. TGD Cobb Salad

MAKES 1 SERVING

INGREDIENTS:

- 2 cups chopped romaine lettuce
- 3 oz grilled chicken breast, diced
- 1 hard-boiled egg, sliced
- ¼ avocado, diced
- 2 slices nitrate-free bacon, cooked and crumbled

- ¼ cup cherry tomatoes, halved
- 1 tablespoon olive oil
- 1 teaspoon red wine vinegar

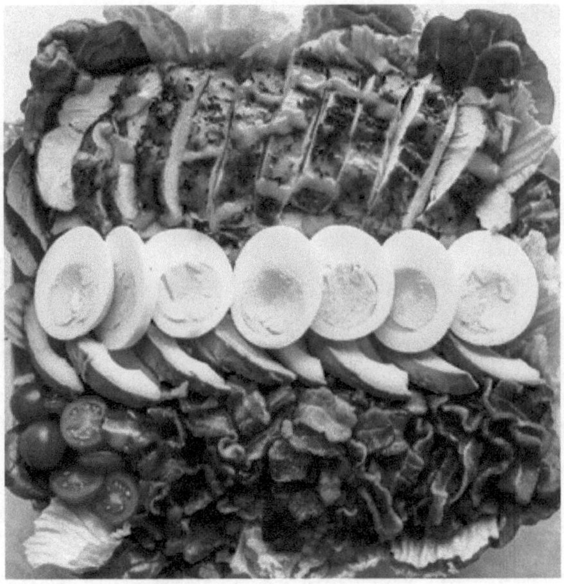

Salt and black pepper to taste

INSTRUCTIONS:

1. Arrange romaine on a plate.
2. Top with chicken, egg, avocado, bacon, and cherry tomatoes in rows or mixed.
3. In a small bowl, whisk olive oil and vinegar with salt and pepper.
4. Drizzle dressing over salad and toss gently.

A classic Cobb made Galveston-style: high protein, healthy fat, and satisfying crunch with no blood sugar spikes.

26. Grape Tomato and Pea Salad on Ricotta Spread

MAKES 1 SERVING

INGREDIENTS:

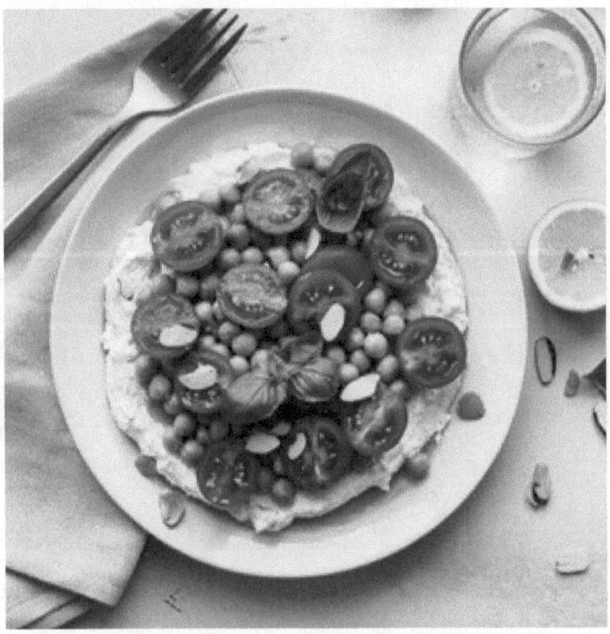

- ¼ cup full-fat ricotta cheese
- ½ cup grape tomatoes, halved
- ¼ cup fresh peas, blanched
- 1 tablespoon olive oil
- 1 teaspoon lemon juice
- 1 teaspoon chopped fresh basil
- ¼ teaspoon ground turmeric
- Salt and black pepper to taste
- 1 tablespoon sliced almonds

INSTRUCTIONS:

1. Spread ricotta cheese evenly onto a plate as a base.
2. In a small bowl, mix grape tomatoes, peas, olive oil, lemon juice, basil, turmeric, salt, and pepper.
3. Spoon the tomato-pea mixture over the ricotta.
4. Sprinkle with sliced almonds.
5. Serve immediately.

This fresh and vibrant lunch balances creamy dairy, fiber-rich vegetables, and anti-inflammatory spices for a light but filling meal.

27. Vegan Protein Salad

MAKES 1 SERVING

INGREDIENTS:

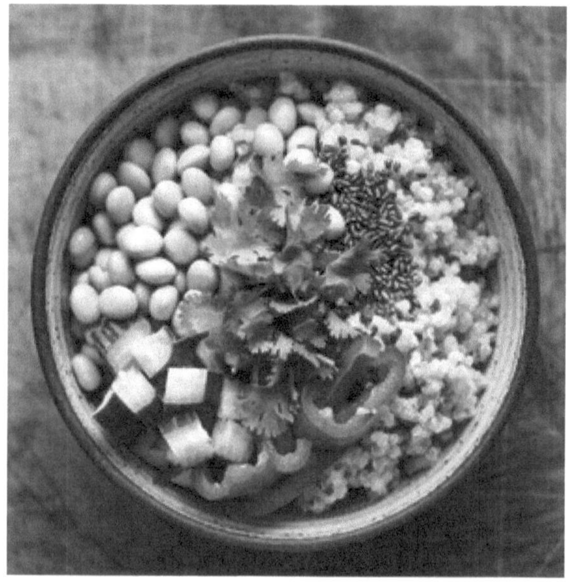

- ½ cup cooked quinoa
- ¼ cup shelled edamame
- ¼ cup diced cucumber
- ¼ cup diced red bell pepper
- 1 tablespoon chia seeds
- 1 tablespoon olive oil
- 1 teaspoon lime juice
- ½ teaspoon ground cumin
- Salt and black pepper to taste
- 1 tablespoon chopped fresh cilantro

INSTRUCTIONS:

1. Combine quinoa, edamame, cucumber, bell pepper, and chia seeds in a bowl.
2. In a small bowl, whisk olive oil, lime juice, cumin, salt, and pepper.
3. Pour dressing over salad and toss well.
4. Garnish with fresh cilantro.
5. Serve immediately or chill for 10 minutes to blend flavors.

This plant-based salad delivers fiber, healthy fats, and protein, making it a colorful, hormone-friendly lunch option.

28. Chicken Taco Salad

MAKES 1 SERVING

INGREDIENTS:

- 3 oz grilled chicken breast, shredded
- 2 cups chopped romaine lettuce
- ¼ cup diced tomatoes

- ¼ avocado, sliced
- 1 tablespoon olive oil
- 1 teaspoon lime juice
- ½ teaspoon chili powder
- ¼ teaspoon ground cumin
- Salt and black pepper to taste
- 1 tablespoon crumbled feta cheese

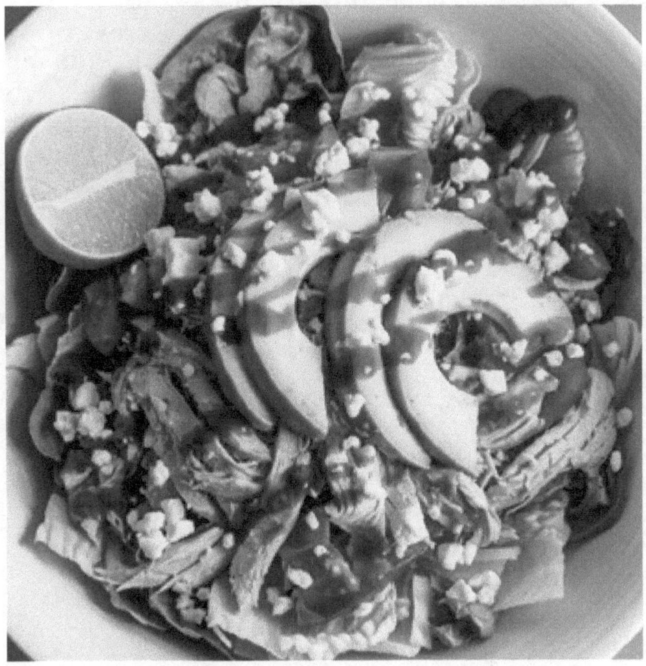

INSTRUCTIONS:

1. Arrange chopped romaine on a plate.
2. Top with chicken, tomatoes, and avocado slices.
3. In a small bowl, whisk olive oil, lime juice, chili powder, cumin, salt, and pepper.
4. Drizzle dressing over the salad.
5. Sprinkle with feta cheese and serve.

This spicy, satisfying taco salad delivers protein, flavor, and healthy fats without any grains or added sugar.

29. Tuna Salad over Mixed Greens

MAKES 1 SERVING

INGREDIENTS:

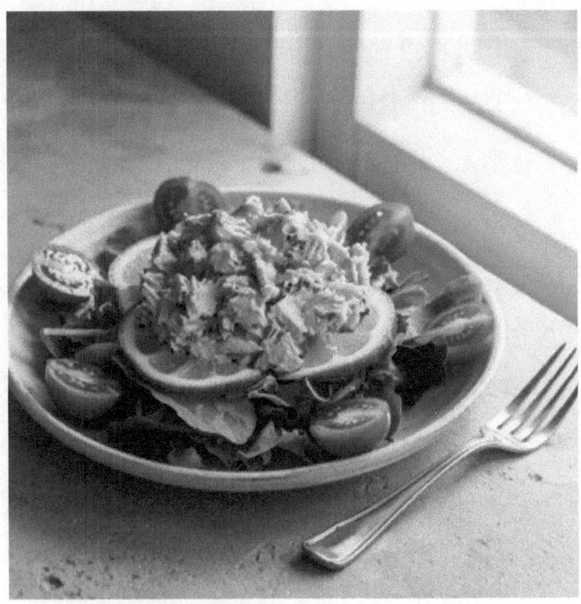

- 1 can (5 oz) tuna in water, drained
- 1 tablespoon olive oil mayonnaise
- 1 teaspoon lemon juice
- ¼ cup diced cucumber
- 2 cups mixed greens (e.g., spinach, arugula)
- ¼ cup cherry tomatoes, halved
- 1 tablespoon olive oil
- ½ teaspoon Dijon mustard
- Salt and black pepper to taste

INSTRUCTIONS:

1. In a bowl, combine tuna, mayonnaise, lemon juice, and cucumber. Season to taste.

2. Arrange greens and cherry tomatoes on a plate.
3. Spoon tuna mixture over the greens.
4. In a small bowl, whisk olive oil and Dijon mustard with salt and pepper.
5. Drizzle dressing over the top and serve.

This low-carb lunch is rich in protein, fiber, and flavor, ideal for hormone balance and sustained energy.

30. Egg and Vegetable Salad

MAKES 1 SERVING

INGREDIENTS:

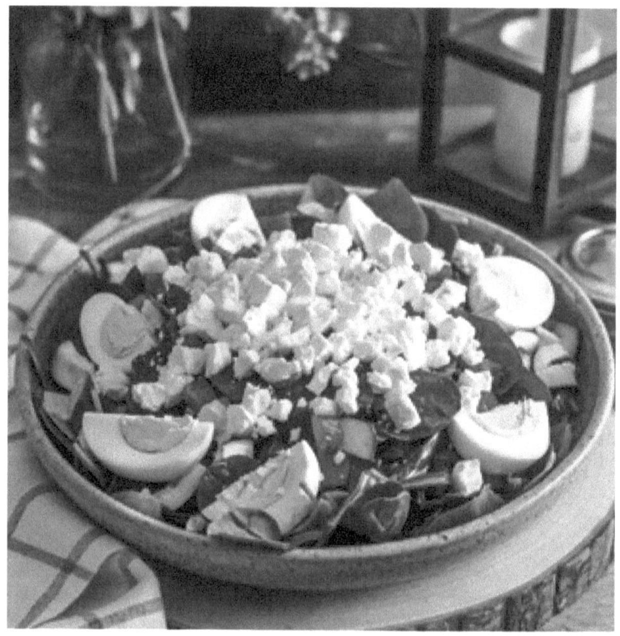

- 2 large eggs, hard-boiled and chopped
- ¼ cup diced zucchini
- ¼ cup diced red bell pepper
- 2 cups baby spinach
- 1 tablespoon olive oil
- 1 teaspoon red wine vinegar
- ¼ teaspoon dried oregano
- Salt and black pepper to taste
- 1 tablespoon crumbled goat cheese

INSTRUCTIONS:

1. In a bowl, combine chopped eggs, zucchini, red bell pepper, and spinach.
2. In a small bowl, whisk olive oil, red wine vinegar, oregano, salt, and pepper.
3. Pour dressing over the salad and toss gently.
4. Sprinkle with goat cheese and serve.

This protein-rich salad combines healthy fats and leafy greens with flavorful veggies and tangy goat cheese for a complete, nourishing meal.

31. Grilled Chicken Salad

MAKES 1 SERVING

INGREDIENTS:

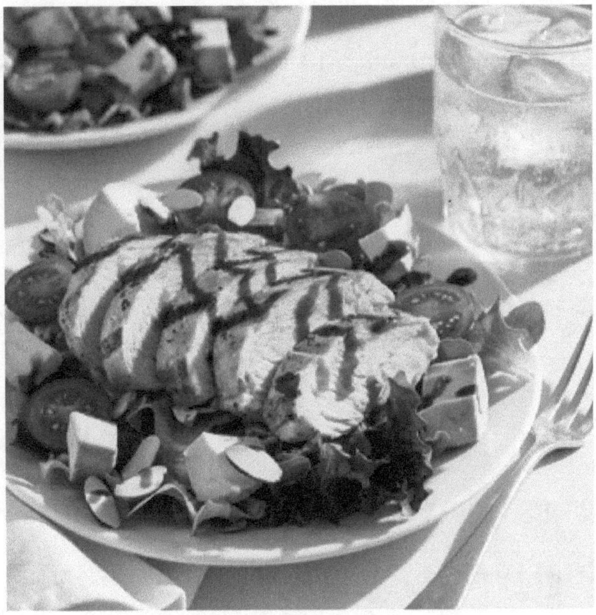

- 3 oz grilled chicken breast, sliced
- 2 cups mixed greens (e.g., arugula, spinach)
- ¼ cup cherry tomatoes, halved
- ¼ avocado, diced
- 1 tablespoon olive oil
- 1 teaspoon balsamic vinegar
- ½ teaspoon Dijon mustard
- Salt and black pepper to taste
- 1 tablespoon sliced almonds

INSTRUCTIONS:

1. Arrange mixed greens on a plate.
2. Top with grilled chicken, cherry tomatoes, and avocado.
3. In a small bowl, whisk olive oil, balsamic vinegar, Dijon mustard, salt, and pepper.
4. Drizzle the dressing over the salad.
5. Sprinkle with sliced almonds and serve immediately.

This Galveston Diet–compliant salad offers protein, healthy fats, and fresh flavor in a quick, energizing meal.

32. Sirloin, Spinach, and Blue Cheese Salad with Pecans

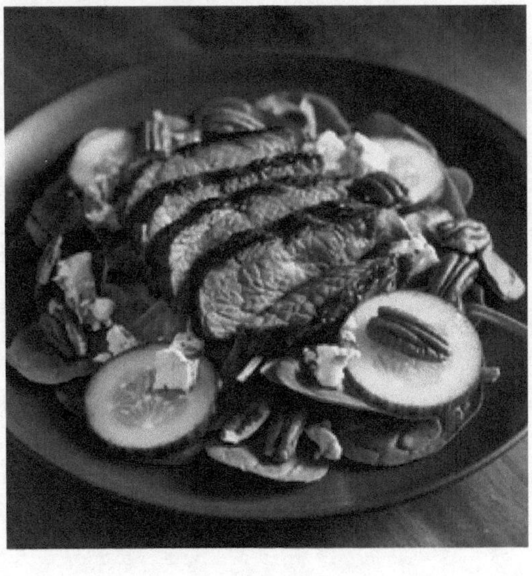

MAKES 1 SERVING

INGREDIENTS:

- 3 oz grilled sirloin steak, thinly sliced
- 2 cups baby spinach
- ¼ cup cucumber, sliced
- 1 tablespoon crumbled blue cheese
- 1 tablespoon chopped pecans
- 1 tablespoon olive oil
- 1 teaspoon red wine vinegar

- ¼ teaspoon dried thyme
- Salt and black pepper to taste

INSTRUCTIONS:

1. Place spinach on a plate and top with sliced steak, cucumber, blue cheese, and pecans.
2. In a small bowl, whisk olive oil, red wine vinegar, thyme, salt, and pepper.
3. Drizzle the dressing over the salad.
4. Toss gently or serve as a composed salad.

This salad is rich in protein, iron, and omega-3s, with tangy blue cheese and earthy greens for balance.

33. Edamame Mash Salad

MAKES 1 SERVING

INGREDIENTS:

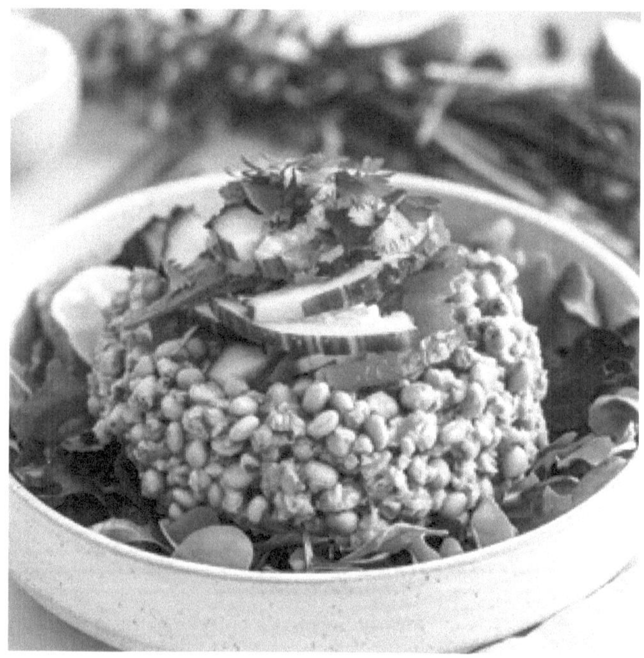

- ½ cup shelled edamame, steamed
- ¼ cup diced cucumber
- ¼ cup diced red bell pepper
- 1 tablespoon olive oil
- 1 teaspoon lime juice
- ½ teaspoon ground cumin
- Salt and black pepper to taste
- 1 tablespoon chopped fresh cilantro
- 2 cups mixed greens

INSTRUCTIONS:

1. In a bowl, mash steamed edamame with a fork until chunky.
2. Mix in cucumber, bell pepper, olive oil, lime juice, cumin, salt, and pepper.
3. Stir in chopped cilantro.
4. Serve the mash over a bed of mixed greens and enjoy immediately.

This high-fiber, high-protein salad is completely plant-based and keeps you full while supporting hormone health.

34. Turkey and Mayo Lettuce Wraps

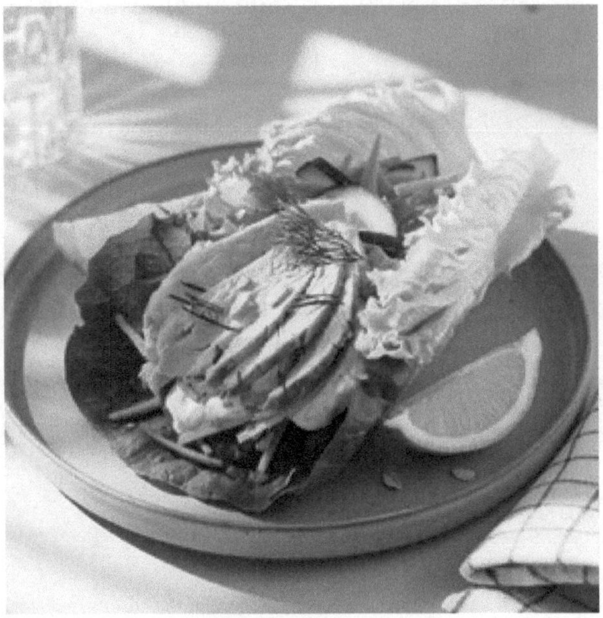

MAKES 1 SERVING

INGREDIENTS:

- 3 oz nitrate-free turkey breast, sliced
- 1 large romaine lettuce leaf
- 1 tablespoon olive oil mayonnaise
- ¼ cup diced cucumber
- ¼ cup shredded carrots
- 1 teaspoon chopped fresh dill
- Salt and black pepper to taste
- 1 tablespoon sliced almonds

INSTRUCTIONS:

1. Lay the lettuce leaf flat and spread mayonnaise in the center.
2. Layer turkey, cucumber, and carrots on top.
3. Sprinkle with dill, salt, and pepper.
4. Add sliced almonds for crunch.
5. Fold the lettuce leaf around the filling and serve immediately.

This wrap delivers satisfying protein and crunch without any grains or added sugar.

35. Naked Turkey Roll-Ups

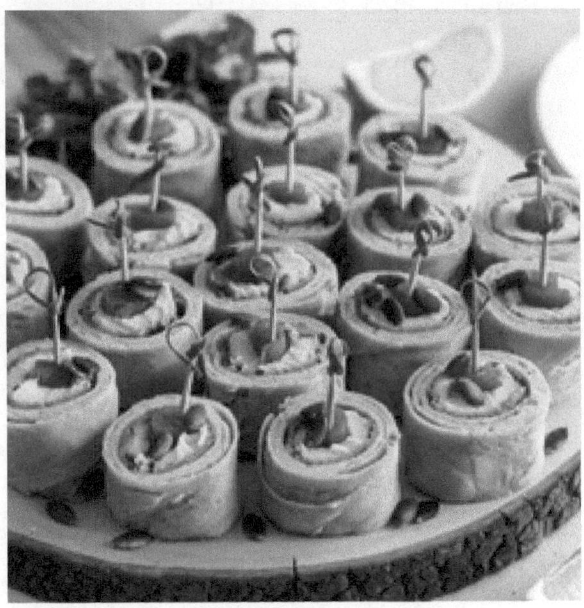

MAKES 1 SERVING

INGREDIENTS:

- 3 oz nitrate-free turkey breast, thinly sliced
- ¼ avocado, mashed
- 1 teaspoon Dijon mustard
- ¼ cup diced red bell pepper
- 1 tablespoon chopped fresh parsley
- Salt and black pepper to taste
- 1 tablespoon pumpkin seeds

INSTRUCTIONS:

1. Spread mashed avocado and mustard over each turkey slice.
2. Sprinkle with bell pepper, parsley, salt, and pepper.
3. Roll up each slice tightly and secure with a toothpick if needed.
4. Sprinkle pumpkin seeds on top or serve alongside.
5. Serve immediately with mixed greens if desired.

These quick roll-ups are protein-rich, full of flavor, and perfect as a snack or light lunch.

36. Hard-Boiled Egg with Avocado

MAKES 1 SERVING

INGREDIENTS:

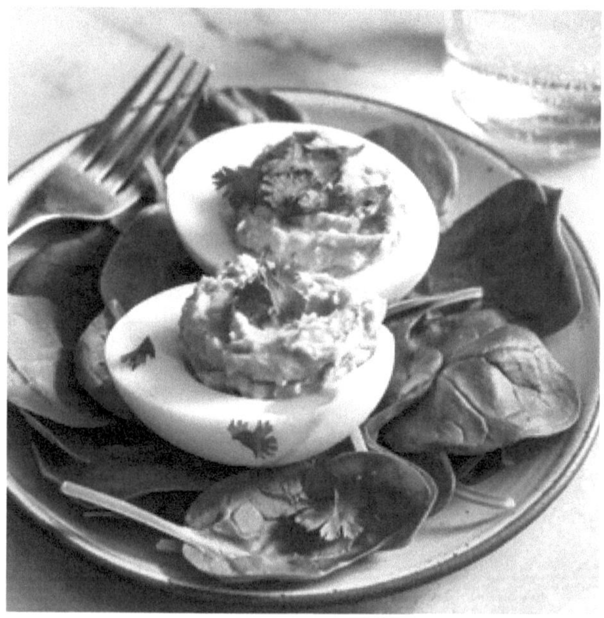

- 2 large eggs, hard-boiled
- ½ avocado, mashed
- 1 teaspoon lime juice
- ¼ teaspoon ground cumin
- Salt and black pepper to taste
- 1 tablespoon chopped fresh cilantro
- 2 cups baby spinach
- 1 tablespoon olive oil

INSTRUCTIONS:

1. Peel and halve the hard-boiled eggs.
2. In a small bowl, mix mashed avocado with lime juice, cumin, salt, and pepper.
3. Spoon the avocado mixture over the egg halves.
4. Arrange baby spinach on a plate and drizzle with olive oil.
5. Place avocado-topped eggs on top of the greens.
6. Sprinkle with cilantro and serve immediately.

This snack or light breakfast is rich in protein and healthy fats, perfect for satiety and hormone support.

III. Clean & Satisfying Dinners

Supports: Evening satiety, cortisol balance, belly fat reduction, and natural hormone support

37. Sesame Ginger Pork with Green Beans

MAKES 1 SERVING

INGREDIENTS:

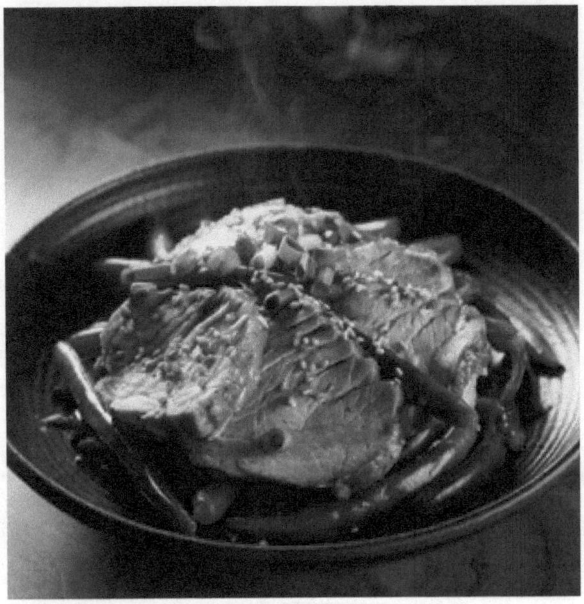

- 4 oz pork tenderloin, thinly sliced
- 1 cup green beans, trimmed
- 1 tablespoon olive oil
- 1 teaspoon sesame oil
- 1 teaspoon grated fresh ginger
- 1 teaspoon coconut aminos
- ½ teaspoon sesame seeds
- Salt and black pepper to taste
- 1 tablespoon chopped green onions

INSTRUCTIONS:

1. Heat olive oil in a skillet over medium heat.
2. Add pork, season with salt and pepper, and cook 3–4 minutes per side until done. Remove and set aside.
3. Add green beans to the same skillet and sauté 5–6 minutes.
4. Stir in sesame oil, ginger, and coconut aminos.
5. Return pork to the skillet and toss to coat.
6. Sprinkle with sesame seeds and green onions and serve.

This protein-rich dish is quick, savory, and compliant with an anti-inflammatory lifestyle.

38. Bell Peppers Stuffed with Turkey and Cauliflower Rice

MAKES 1 SERVING

INGREDIENTS:

- 1 large red bell pepper, halved and seeded
- 4 oz ground nitrate-free turkey
- ½ cup cauliflower rice

- ¼ cup diced tomatoes
- 1 tablespoon olive oil
- ½ teaspoon ground cumin
- ¼ teaspoon smoked paprika
- Salt and black pepper to taste
- 1 tablespoon chopped fresh cilantro

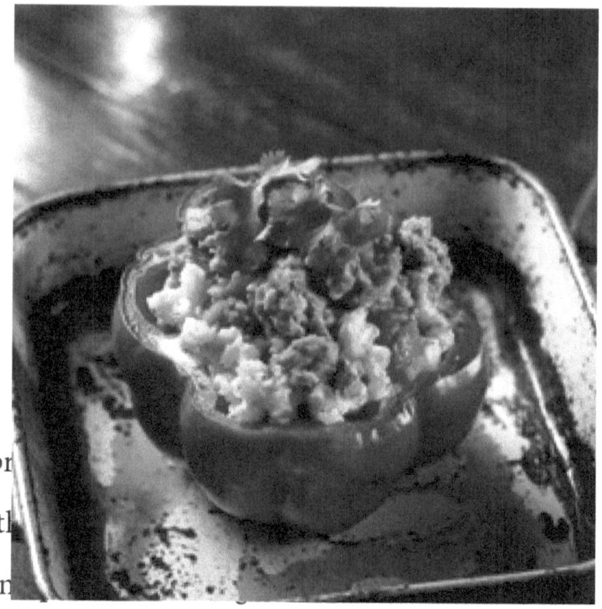

INSTRUCTIONS:

1. Preheat oven to 375°F.
2. Heat olive oil in a skillet. Add turkey, cumin, papr
3. Add cauliflower rice and tomatoes and cook anot
4. Stuff the pepper halves with the turkey mixture ar
5. Bake for 20–25 minutes until peppers are tender.
6. Garnish with cilantro and serve.

A flavorful, grain-free, fiber-filled dinner option packed with lean protein and veggies.

39. Shrimp and Asparagus

MAKES 1 SERVING

INGREDIENTS:

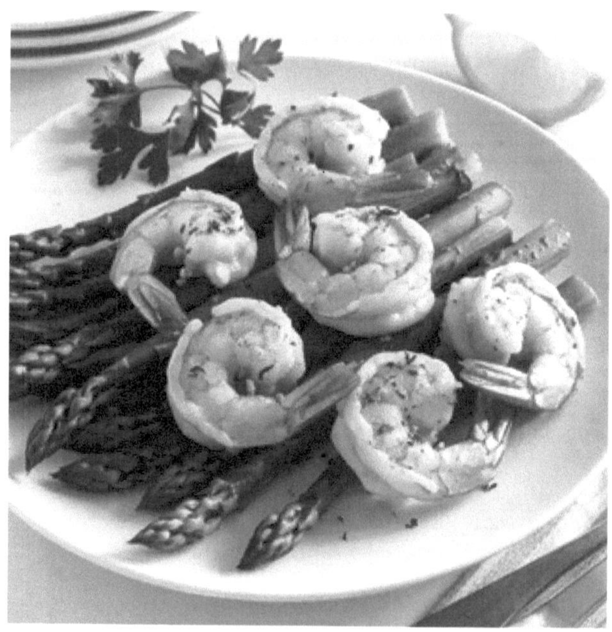

- 4 oz large shrimp, peeled and deveined
- 1 cup asparagus spears, trimmed
- 1 tablespoon olive oil
- 1 teaspoon lemon juice
- ½ teaspoon garlic powder
- ¼ teaspoon smoked paprika
- Salt and black pepper to taste
- 1 tablespoon chopped fresh parsley

INSTRUCTIONS:

1. Heat olive oil in a skillet over medium heat.
2. Season shrimp with garlic powder, paprika, salt, and pepper. Cook 2–3 minutes per side. Remove and set aside.
3. Add asparagus to the skillet and cook for 5–6 minutes until tender-crisp.

4. Drizzle with lemon juice and season as needed.
5. Return shrimp to the pan and toss together.
6. Sprinkle with parsley and serve hot.

This dish is low in carbs and high in protein, with refreshing lemon and spice for flavor.

40. Pumpkin and Chicken Curry with Cauliflower Rice

MAKES 1 SERVING

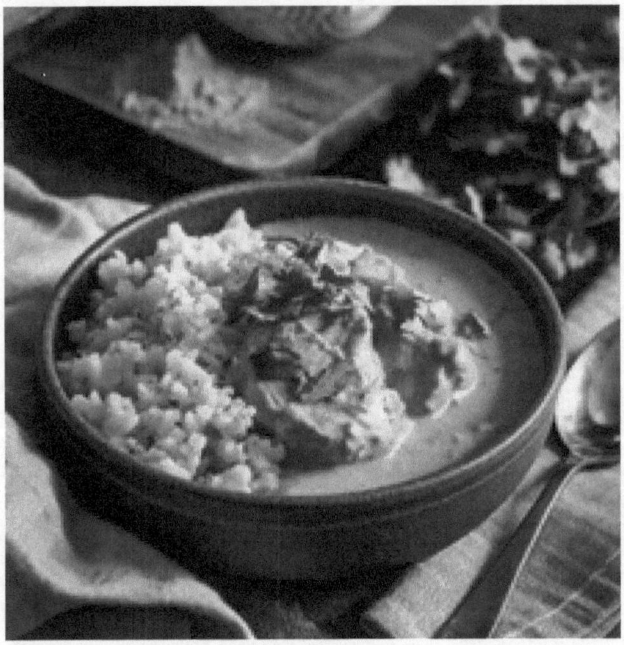

INGREDIENTS:

- 4 oz chicken breast, diced
- ½ cup pumpkin puree
- ½ cup cauliflower rice
- 1 tablespoon coconut oil
- ½ teaspoon curry powder
- ¼ teaspoon ground turmeric
- ¼ cup unsweetened coconut milk
- Salt and black pepper to taste
- 1 tablespoon chopped fresh cilantro

INSTRUCTIONS:

1. Heat coconut oil in a skillet over medium heat.
2. Add chicken, curry powder, turmeric, salt, and pepper. Cook 5–6 minutes until browned.
3. Stir in pumpkin puree and coconut milk. Simmer for 5 minutes until thickened.
4. In another skillet, sauté cauliflower rice with salt for 3–4 minutes.
5. Serve curry over cauliflower rice.
6. Garnish with cilantro and enjoy.

A warm, anti-inflammatory meal combining protein, fiber, and comforting spices for a satisfying dinner.

41. Tofu in Peanut Sauce

MAKES 1 SERVING

INGREDIENTS:

- 4 oz firm tofu, cubed

- 1 tablespoon no-sugar-added peanut butter
- 1 teaspoon coconut aminos
- ½ teaspoon grated fresh ginger
- 1 tablespoon olive oil
- ½ cup broccoli florets
- ¼ cup diced red bell pepper
- Salt and black pepper to taste
- 1 tablespoon chopped green onions

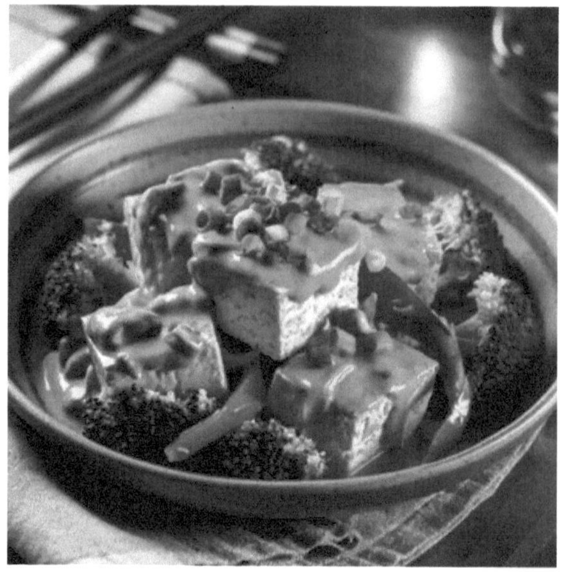

INSTRUCTIONS:

1. In a small bowl, whisk peanut butter, coconut aminos, ginger, and 1 tablespoon water to make a sauce.
2. Heat olive oil in a skillet over medium heat.
3. Add tofu, season with salt and pepper, and cook for 5–6 minutes until golden. Remove and set aside.
4. In the same skillet, sauté broccoli and bell pepper for 5 minutes until tender-crisp.
5. Return tofu to the skillet and pour in peanut sauce. Stir to coat.
6. Garnish with chopped green onions and serve hot.

This vegan-friendly dish delivers plant-based protein, healthy fats, and anti-inflammatory ingredients in one savory meal.

42. Portobello Pizzas

MAKES 1 SERVING

INGREDIENTS:

- 2 large portobello mushroom caps, stems removed
- 4 oz ground nitrate-free turkey
- ¼ cup no-sugar-added marinara sauce
- 1 tablespoon olive oil
- ¼ cup shredded mozzarella cheese
- ¼ cup diced green bell pepper
- ½ teaspoon dried oregano
- Salt and black pepper to taste

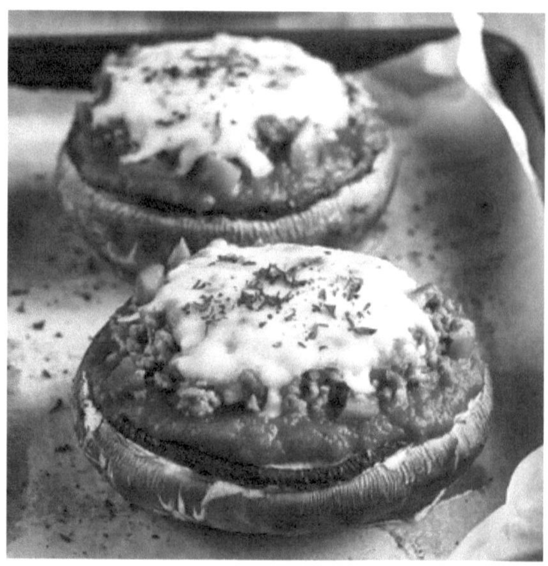

INSTRUCTIONS:

1. Preheat oven to 400°F.
2. Brush mushroom caps with olive oil and bake for 5 minutes.
3. In a skillet, cook ground turkey with salt, pepper, and oregano until browned.
4. Spread marinara sauce onto the mushrooms.
5. Top with cooked turkey, bell pepper, and shredded cheese.
6. Bake for 10–12 minutes until cheese is melted.
7. Serve warm, optionally with a side salad.

A delicious low-carb pizza alternative that's rich in protein and healthy fats.

43. Cheeseburger Lettuce Sliders

MAKES 1 SERVING

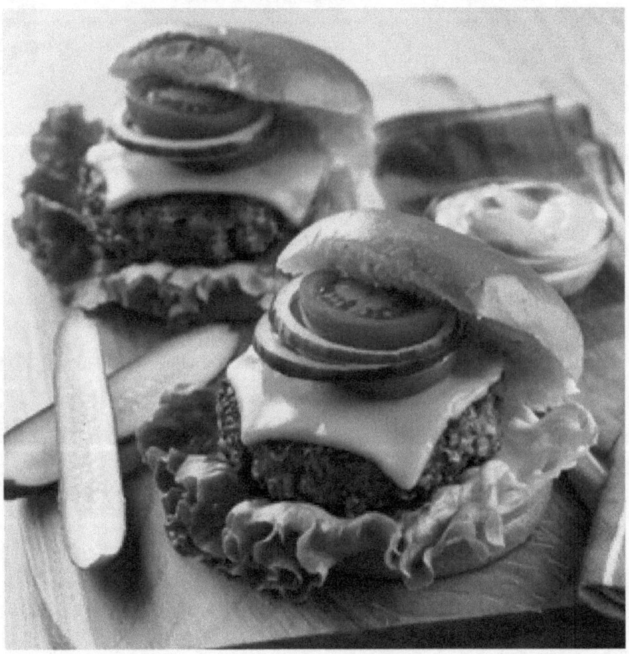

INGREDIENTS:

- 4 oz ground grass-fed beef
- 2 large romaine lettuce leaves
- 1 tablespoon olive oil mayonnaise
- ¼ cup sliced cherry tomatoes
- 1 slice cheddar cheese
- ¼ teaspoon garlic powder
- Salt and black pepper to taste
- 1 tablespoon chopped red onion

INSTRUCTIONS:

1. Form ground beef into two small patties.
2. Season with garlic powder, salt, and pepper.
3. Cook in a skillet over medium heat for 3–4 minutes per side.
4. During the last minute, place cheese on one patty to melt.
5. Place each patty on a lettuce leaf.
6. Top with mayonnaise, tomatoes, and red onion.
7. Fold lettuce into sliders and serve immediately.

These sliders are low in carbs and high in flavor, making them a satisfying Galveston-approved meal.

44. BLT Salmon Burgers

MAKES 4 SERVINGS

INGREDIENTS:

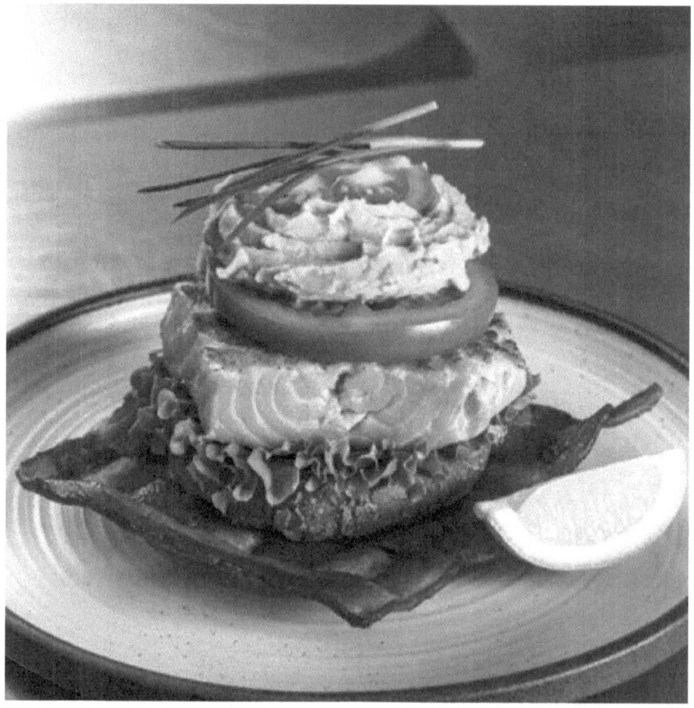

- 16 slices turkey bacon, halved
- 1 (8 oz) poached salmon fillet, skin removed
- 2–3 tablespoons mayonnaise
- Salt and black pepper
- 2 tablespoons olive oil
- 2 avocados, mashed
- 4 tablespoons ground flaxseed
- Juice of ½ lemon
- 3 tablespoons minced fresh chives
- 4 butter lettuce leaves
- 4 slices ripe tomato

INSTRUCTIONS:

1. Preheat oven to 400°F. Weave bacon into 4 flat squares and bake 25 minutes until crisp.
2. Mash salmon with mayonnaise and season with salt and pepper. Form into patties.
3. Heat olive oil in a skillet and cook patties 4 minutes per side.
4. Mix mashed avocado with flaxseed, lemon juice, and chives.
5. Assemble each "bun" with a bacon weave base, avocado mash, salmon patty, lettuce, and tomato.
6. Serve open-faced or top with another bacon weave.

High in protein and omega-3s, these savory burgers are a fun, nutrient-dense meal.

45. Baked Salmon with Grilled Summer Squash

MAKES 4 SERVINGS

INGREDIENTS (Squash):

- 1 yellow squash, sliced
- 1 zucchini, sliced
- 1 tablespoon melted unsalted butter
- 1 lemon, zested and juiced

- Salt, black pepper, and cayenne to taste

INGREDIENTS (Salmon):

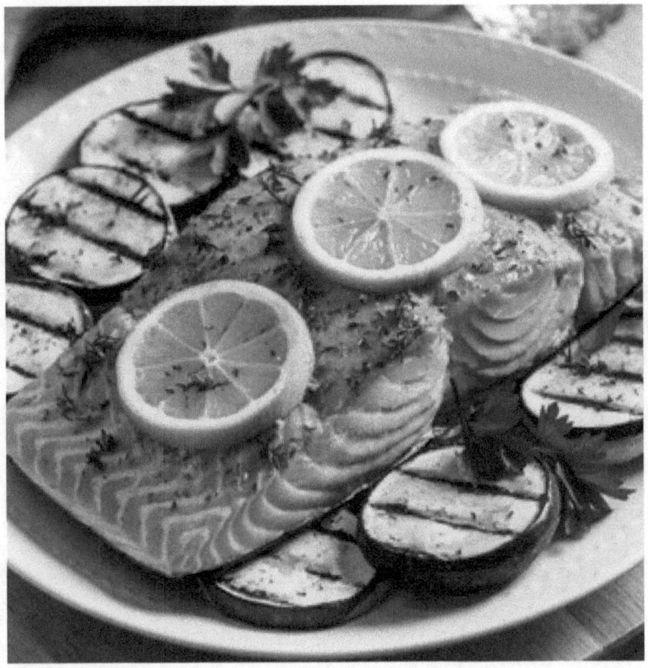

- 1 large salmon fillet (about 3 lbs)
- Salt and black pepper
- 6 tablespoons melted butter
- 1 tablespoon honey
- 3 garlic cloves, minced
- 1 teaspoon chopped thyme
- 1 teaspoon dried oregano
- 1 lemon, thinly sliced
- Fresh parsley, for garnish

INSTRUCTIONS:

1. Preheat grill to medium. Toss squash with butter, lemon zest, juice, and seasoning. Wrap in foil and grill for 30 minutes.
2. Preheat oven to 350°F. Line a baking sheet with foil.
3. Place lemon slices on foil and set salmon on top.
4. Mix melted butter, honey, garlic, thyme, and oregano and pour over salmon.
5. Fold foil and bake 15–20 minutes. Broil 2 minutes until golden.
6. Serve salmon with grilled squash and garnish with parsley.

A beautiful, hormone-friendly meal that combines lean protein with antioxidant-rich veggies and herbs.

46. Grilled Shrimp with Broiled Tomato Bites

MAKES 4 SERVINGS

INGREDIENTS (Shrimp):

- ⅓ cup olive oil
- 2 tablespoons lemon juice
- 1 teaspoon salt
- ¼ teaspoon black pepper
- 1 teaspoon Italian seasoning
- 2 teaspoons minced garlic
- 1 lb large shrimp, peeled and deveined

- 4 bamboo skewers
- Fresh parsley and lemon wedges for garnish

INGREDIENTS (Tomatoes):

- 8 small tomatoes
- 2 tablespoons olive oil
- ¼ cup grated Parmesan
- Nonstick cooking spray

INSTRUCTIONS:

1. In a bowl, whisk oil, lemon juice, salt, pepper, seasoning, and garlic. Add shrimp and marinate 15 minutes.
2. Soak skewers in water. Thread shrimp onto skewers.
3. Grill shrimp over medium heat for 2–3 minutes per side.
4. Halve tomatoes and trim bottoms so they sit flat. Place in a greased baking dish.
5. Brush with olive oil, sprinkle with Parmesan, and broil for 3 minutes.
6. Serve shrimp skewers with broiled tomatoes. Garnish with parsley and lemon.

A vibrant, high-protein meal with minimal carbs and tons of fresh flavor.

47. Lemon Chicken with Capers

MAKES 4 SERVINGS

INGREDIENTS:

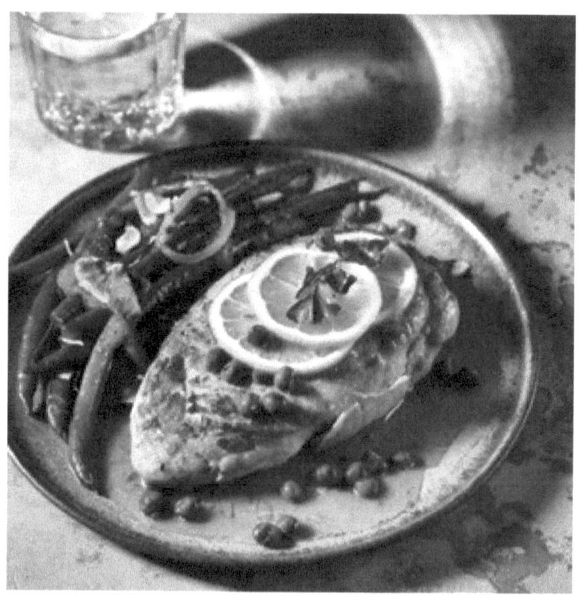

- 4 boneless chicken breasts
- Salt and pepper
- 4 tablespoons ghee or olive oil
- 2 lemons (1 juiced, 1 sliced)
- 1 garlic clove, sliced
- 2 tablespoons capers
- 1 large onion, sliced
- 4 cups green beans
- ¼ cup toasted slivered almonds

INSTRUCTIONS:

1. Season chicken with salt and pepper. In a skillet, heat 1 tbsp ghee and cook chicken until done.

Remove and keep warm.

2. In the same pan, add lemon juice, 1 tbsp ghee, garlic, capers, and lemon slices. Simmer and return chicken to coat.

3. In another skillet, sauté onion and green beans in 2 tbsp ghee until tender.

4. Toss beans with almonds.

5. Serve chicken with lemon-caper sauce and a side of green beans.

Bright, zesty, and protein-rich, this dish supports hormone balance and digestion.

48. Broccoli and Cheese Chicken Bake

MAKES 4 SERVINGS

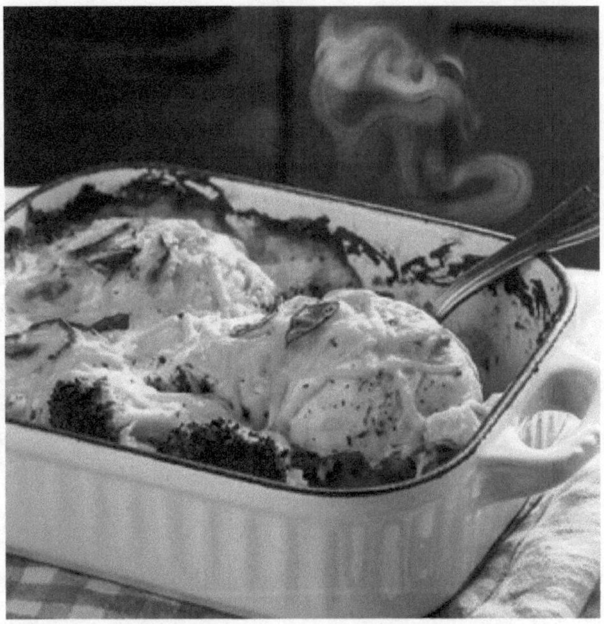

INGREDIENTS:

- 3 cups cooked chopped chicken breast
- 4 cups cooked broccoli florets
- 2 tablespoons olive oil
- ½ cup sour cream
- ½ cup heavy cream
- 1 garlic clove, minced
- 1 teaspoon minced basil
- Salt and black pepper to taste
- 1 cup shredded cheddar cheese

INSTRUCTIONS:

1. Preheat oven to 375°F.

2. In a casserole dish, toss chicken and broccoli with olive oil.

3. In a bowl, mix sour cream, heavy cream, garlic, basil, salt, and pepper. Pour over chicken and broccoli.

4. Sprinkle with cheese.

5. Bake for 7–10 minutes until heated through and bubbly.

6. Serve hot.

Comforting, creamy, and hormone-supportive, ideal for batch cooking and leftovers.

49. Spaghetti Squash with Turkey, Bacon, Spinach, and Goat Cheese

MAKES 1 SERVING

INGREDIENTS:

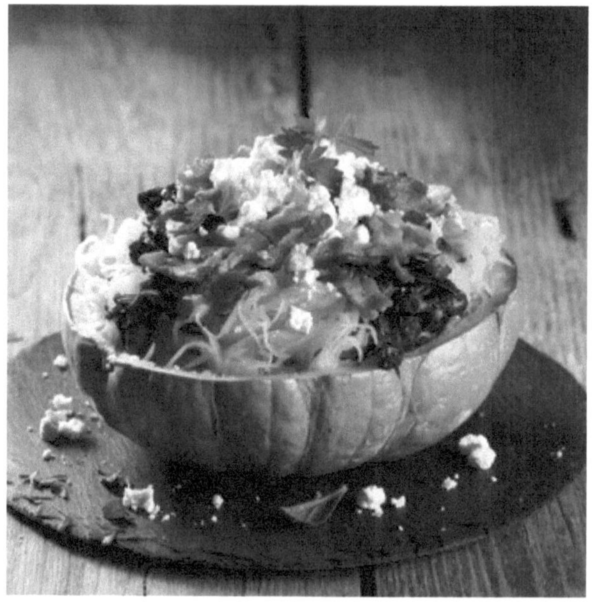

- 1 cup cooked spaghetti squash strands
- 4 oz ground nitrate-free turkey
- 2 slices nitrate-free bacon, chopped
- 1 cup baby spinach
- 1 tablespoon olive oil
- 1 tablespoon crumbled goat cheese
- ½ teaspoon garlic powder
- Salt and black pepper to taste
- 1 tablespoon chopped fresh parsley

INSTRUCTIONS:

1. In a skillet, cook bacon until crisp. Remove and set aside.
2. In the same skillet, cook turkey with garlic powder, salt, and pepper for 5–6 minutes.
3. Add spinach and cook until wilted.
4. Stir in spaghetti squash and bacon.
5. Top with goat cheese and parsley.
6. Serve warm, optionally with cherry tomatoes on the side.

A hearty, low-carb dinner packed with protein and healthy fats.

50. Meatloaf with Cauliflower Mash

MAKES 1 SERVING

INGREDIENTS (Meatloaf):

- 4 oz ground grass-fed beef
- 1 tablespoon ground flaxseed
- 1 tablespoon diced onion
- ½ teaspoon garlic powder
- ¼ teaspoon dried thyme
- Salt and black pepper to taste

INGREDIENTS (Cauliflower Mash):

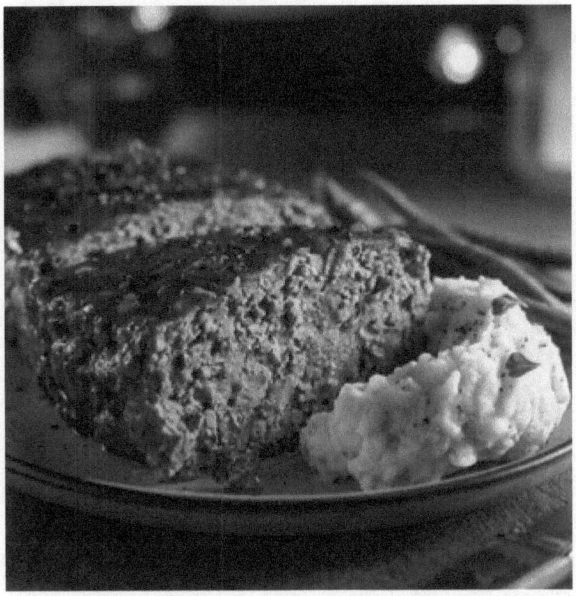

- 1 cup cauliflower florets, steamed
- 1 tablespoon olive oil
- 1 tablespoon full-fat Greek yogurt

INSTRUCTIONS:

1. Preheat oven to 375°F. In a bowl, mix beef, flaxseed, onion, garlic powder, thyme, salt, and pepper.
2. Form into a loaf and place in a baking dish. Bake for 20–25 minutes.
3. In a blender, mix steamed cauliflower, olive oil, Greek yogurt, salt, and pepper until smooth.
4. Serve meatloaf over cauliflower mash.
5. Optional: Add steamed green beans for fiber.

A comforting, low-carb meal with classic flavors and Galveston-friendly ingredients.

51. Grilled Steak with Creamed Spinach and Mushrooms

MAKES 1 SERVING

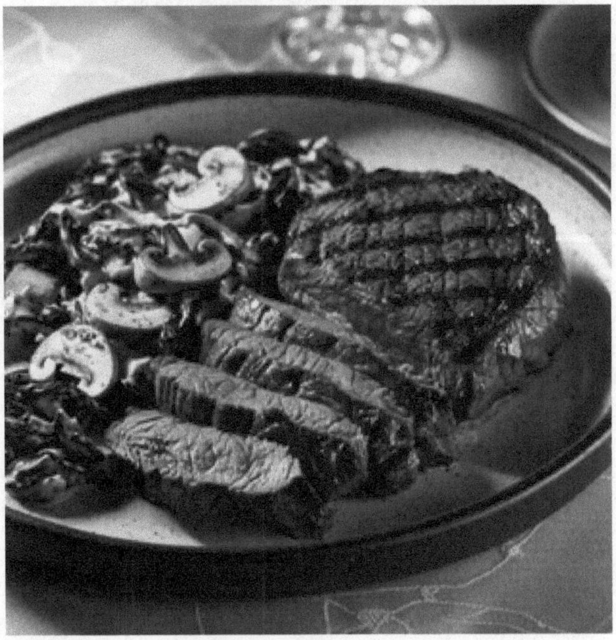

INGREDIENTS:

- 4 oz grass-fed sirloin steak
- 1 cup baby spinach
- ½ cup sliced cremini mushrooms
- 1 tablespoon olive oil
- 1 tablespoon full-fat Greek yogurt
- ½ teaspoon garlic powder
- ¼ teaspoon ground nutmeg
- Salt and black pepper to taste

INSTRUCTIONS:

1. Heat a grill pan over medium-high heat.
2. Season steak with salt, pepper, and ½ tablespoon olive oil. Grill for 3–4 minutes per side. Let rest 5 minutes.
3. In a skillet, heat remaining olive oil and sauté mushrooms for 4–5 minutes.
4. Add spinach, garlic powder, nutmeg, salt, and pepper. Cook until spinach wilts.

5. Stir in Greek yogurt for creaminess.
6. Serve steak with the spinach-mushroom mixture.

A balanced, iron-rich dinner that pairs tender steak with fiber-packed greens and healthy fats.

52. Slow Cooker Mushroom Stroganoff with Creamy Garlic Cauliflower Rice

MAKES 1 SERVING

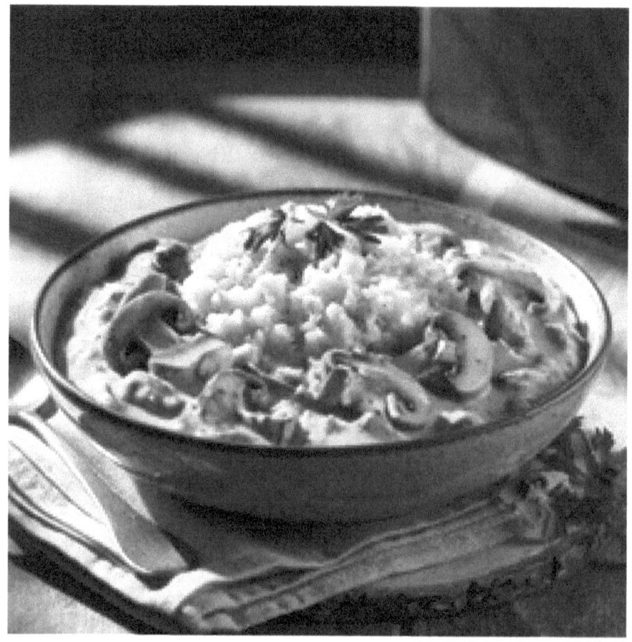

INGREDIENTS:

- 1 cup sliced cremini mushrooms
- ¼ cup diced onion
- 1 tablespoon olive oil
- ¼ cup unsweetened coconut milk
- ½ teaspoon garlic powder
- Salt and black pepper to taste
- 1 cup cauliflower rice
- 1 tablespoon full-fat Greek yogurt
- 1 tablespoon chopped fresh parsley

INSTRUCTIONS:

1. In a slow cooker, combine mushrooms, onion, olive oil, coconut milk, garlic powder, salt, and pepper. Cook on low for 3–4 hours.
2. In a skillet, sauté cauliflower rice with salt and pepper for 3–4 minutes.
3. Stir in Greek yogurt and ¼ teaspoon garlic powder.
4. Serve stroganoff over cauliflower rice.
5. Garnish with parsley and serve warm.

A comforting, creamy vegan-style dinner that's low-carb and gut-friendly.

53. Blackened Tofu with Sesame Broccoli Slaw

MAKES 1 SERVING

INGREDIENTS:

- 4 oz firm tofu, sliced
- 1 cup shredded broccoli slaw (broccoli stems, carrots)

- 1 tablespoon olive oil
- 1 teaspoon sesame oil
- ½ teaspoon blackened seasoning (paprika, cayenne, garlic)
- 1 teaspoon coconut aminos
- Salt and black pepper to taste
- 1 tablespoon sesame seeds

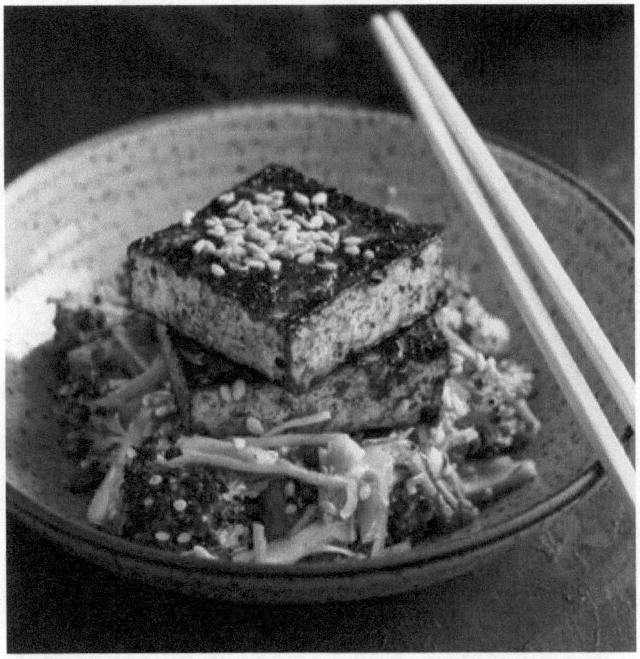

INSTRUCTIONS:

1. Pat tofu dry and coat with blackened seasoning, salt, and pepper.
2. Heat olive oil in a skillet over medium heat. Cook tofu for 3–4 minutes per side until crispy. Remove and set aside.
3. In the same skillet, add broccoli slaw, sesame oil, and coconut aminos. Sauté for 3–4 minutes.
4. Serve tofu over slaw and sprinkle with sesame seeds.

A protein-packed plant-based dinner with crunch, spice, and satisfying fats.

54. BBQ Tempeh, Greens, and Cauliflower Rice

MAKES 4 SERVINGS

INGREDIENTS:

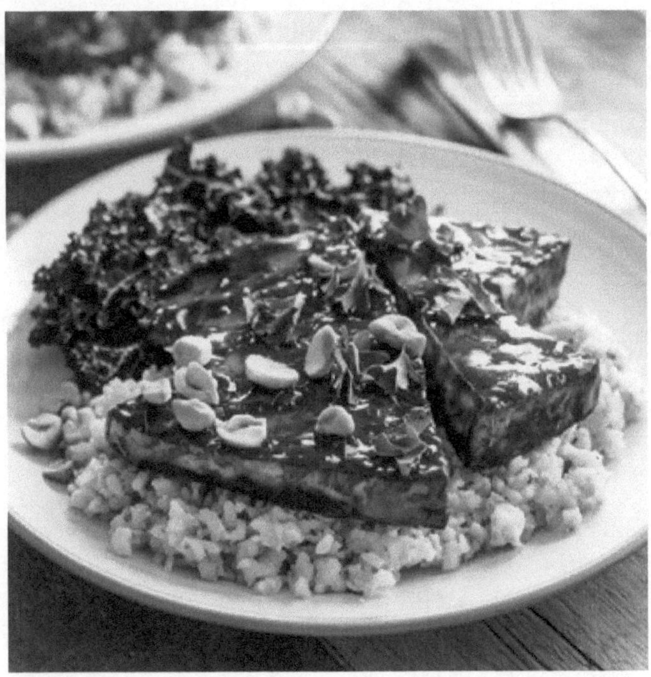

- 2 (8 oz) tempeh blocks, cut into triangles
- ½ cup Primal Kitchen BBQ sauce
- ½ cup orange juice
- 2½ tablespoons tamari
- 2 tablespoons apple cider vinegar
- 1 head cauliflower, riced
- ½ medium onion, diced
- 2 tablespoons ghee
- 1 teaspoon garlic powder
- ¼ teaspoon nutmeg
- Salt and black pepper to taste

- ½ cup chopped parsley
- ½ cup grated Parmesan
- 3 garlic cloves
- 6 cups chopped kale
- 2 tablespoons olive oil
- 2 tablespoons coconut oil
- Roasted peanuts (optional)

INSTRUCTIONS:

1. Marinate tempeh in BBQ sauce, orange juice, tamari, and vinegar for 1 hour.
2. Sauté onion in ghee, add cauliflower rice, garlic powder, nutmeg, salt, and pepper. Cook until tender. Stir in parsley and Parmesan.
3. Sauté kale with olive oil and garlic until wilted.
4. Grill or sear tempeh in coconut oil until golden.
5. Serve tempeh over cauliflower rice and kale. Garnish with leftover marinade and peanuts if using.

A flavor-loaded plant-based meal high in protein, fiber, and healthy fats.

55. Veggie Cheese Enchiladas with Grain-Free Tortillas

MAKES 4 SERVINGS

INGREDIENTS (Tortillas):

- Almond flour, coconut flour, xanthan gum, baking powder, salt
- Lime juice, egg, water

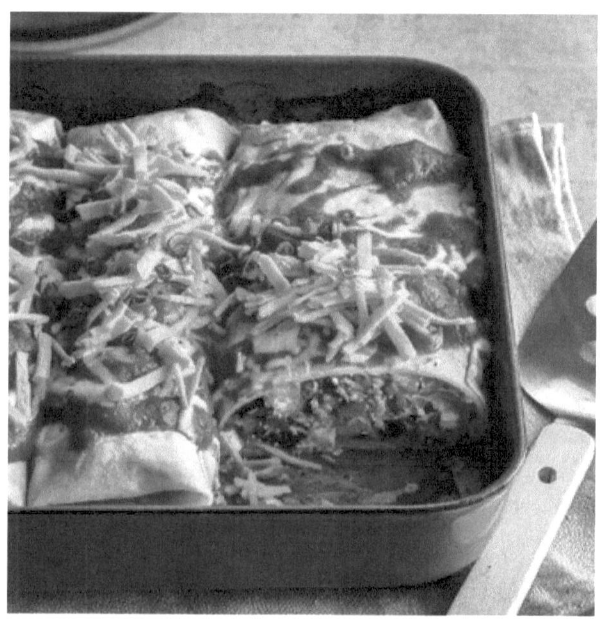

INGREDIENTS (Sauce):

- Tomato sauce, broth, vinegar
- Chili powder, cumin, paprika, garlic/onion powder, salt

INGREDIENTS (Filling):

- Avocado oil
- Onion, bell pepper, zucchini
- Eggs, spinach
- Chili powder, garlic salt, cumin
- 1½ cups shredded cheddar cheese

INSTRUCTIONS:

1. Prepare tortilla dough. Chill, roll, and cook each for 20 seconds per side.
2. Simmer enchilada sauce until thickened.
3. Sauté vegetables, scramble eggs, wilt spinach, and season.
4. Fill each tortilla with veggie-egg mix and cheese. Roll and place in a baking dish.
5. Top with enchilada sauce and extra cheese.
6. Bake at 350°F for 30 minutes. Serve hot.

A hearty, grain-free twist on classic enchiladas, loaded with veggies, eggs, and satisfying spice.

IV. Nourishing Soups & Salads

Supports: Digestive health, inflammation reduction, immune support, and hydration

56. Roasted Tomato Bisque

MAKES 4 SERVINGS

INGREDIENTS:

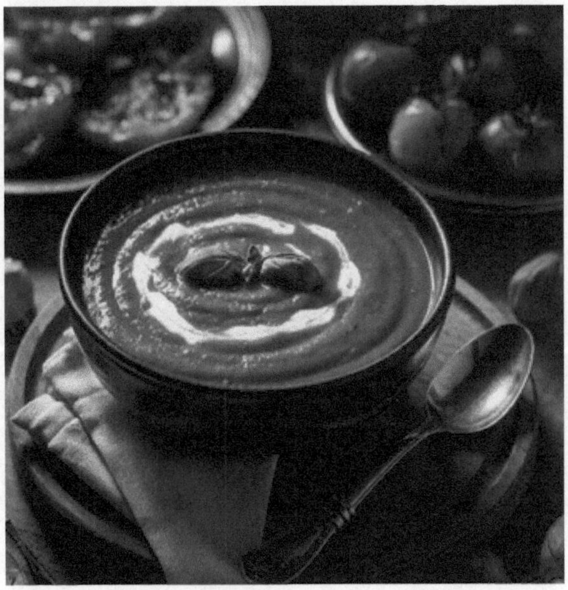

- 8 Roma tomatoes, halved
- 4 garlic cloves
- 4 tbsp olive oil
- 1 (15 oz) can cannellini beans
- 2 cups chicken broth
- Salt and pepper
- 1 cup heavy cream
- Fresh basil (optional)

DIRECTIONS:

1. Roast tomatoes and garlic on a baking sheet at 400°F for 20–25 minutes.
2. Blend with cannellini beans until smooth.
3. In a pot, combine puree with broth. Heat through and season with salt and pepper.
4. Stir in heavy cream and simmer gently.
5. Serve hot, topped with fresh basil if desired. Enjoy with a protein side or salad for a complete meal.

57. Cucumber, Tomato, and Feta Salad

MAKES 1 SERVING

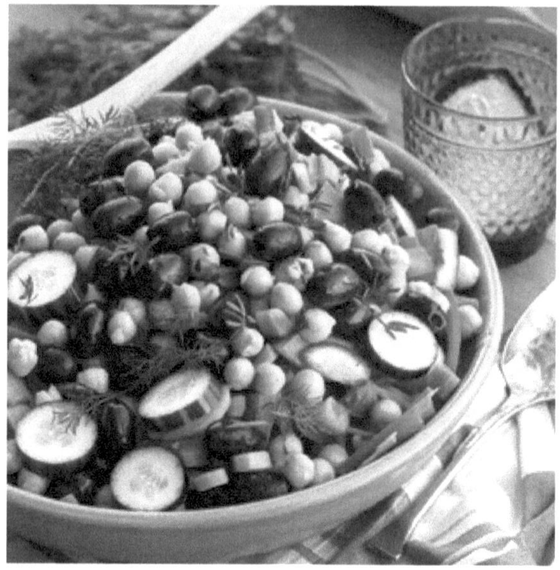

INGREDIENTS:

- 1 medium cucumber, sliced
- 1 cup halved cherry tomatoes
- ¼ small red onion, diced
- 1 garlic clove, minced
- 1 tbsp olive oil
- 1 tbsp red wine vinegar
- 2 tbsp crumbled feta cheese

DIRECTIONS:

1. In a salad bowl, combine cucumber, cherry tomatoes, onion, and garlic.
2. Drizzle with olive oil and red wine vinegar. Toss gently to coat.
3. Sprinkle with feta cheese on top. Serve immediately as a refreshing side or light lunch.
4. This dish pairs well with grilled fish or chicken and is perfect for a warm afternoon.

58. Marinated Olives, Chickpeas, and Vegetables

MAKES 4 SERVINGS

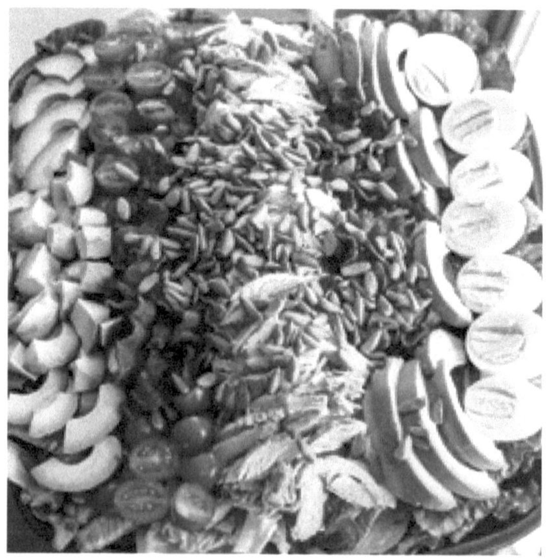

INGREDIENTS:

- 2 large cucumbers, sliced
- 2 medium carrots, sliced
- 1 (15 oz) can chickpeas, drained
- 2 cups olives (any variety)
- ½ cup red wine vinegar
- ¼ cup fresh thyme leaves
- ¼ cup fresh dill

DIRECTIONS:

1. In a large bowl, combine cucumbers, carrots, chickpeas, and olives.
2. Pour in the vinegar and stir in thyme and dill. Toss well.
3. Cover and refrigerate for 15 minutes. Serve chilled.

4. This bright salad works beautifully as a picnic item, lunchbox side, or as a tangy topping on greens or grain bowls.

59. TGD Cobb Salad

MAKES 4 SERVINGS

INGREDIENTS:

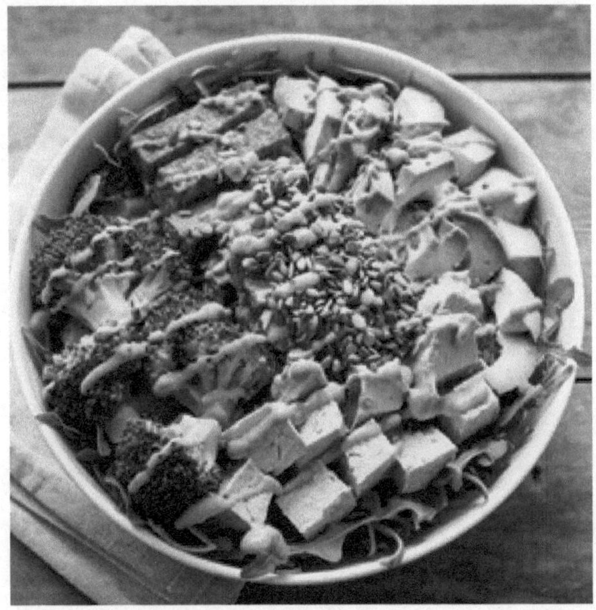

- 8 cups chopped romaine lettuce
- 2 cups shredded cooked chicken
- 12 slices turkey bacon, cooked and chopped
- 2 avocados, chopped
- 8 hard-boiled eggs, quartered
- 1½ cups halved cherry tomatoes
- ½ cup ranch dressing
- 4 tbsp sunflower seeds

DIRECTIONS:

1. In a large bowl, toss romaine with chicken, bacon, avocado, eggs, and tomatoes.
2. Drizzle with ranch and toss gently to coat.
3. Sprinkle with sunflower seeds before serving.
4. This salad can be made ahead and portioned into containers for several meals.

60. Vegan Protein Salad

MAKES 2 SERVINGS

INGREDIENTS:

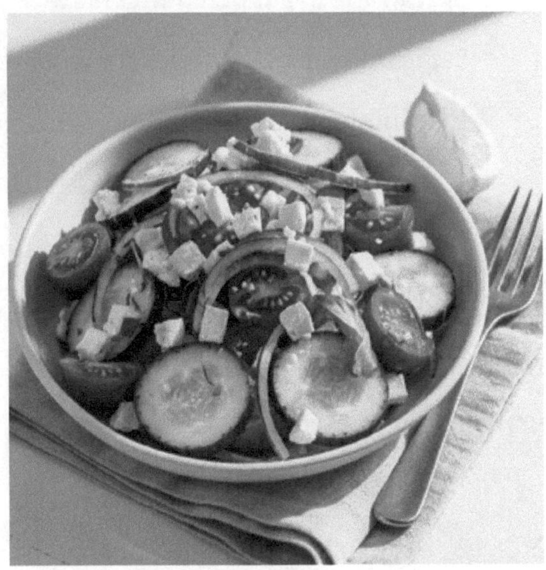

- 4 oz tempeh, marinated in balsamic, tamari, maple, garlic
- 5 oz firm tofu, cubed and baked with garlic and tamari
- 1 cup steamed broccoli
- 2 cups arugula
- 1 cup diced cucumber
- 1 avocado, chopped

- 4 tbsp hemp seeds
- 1 tbsp tahini
- 1 tbsp olive oil
- Lemon juice, to taste

DIRECTIONS:

1. Bake marinated tempeh and tofu at 400°F until browned.
2. In a large bowl, toss broccoli, arugula, cucumber, and avocado.
3. Add baked tempeh and tofu.
4. Drizzle with tahini, olive oil, and lemon juice. Top with hemp seeds.
5. Perfect for meal prep and adaptable to any grain bowl or wrap.

V. Dips, Spreads & Crunchy Bites

Supports: Healthy snacking, mood stability, clean eating, and hormone-friendly fat intake

61. Celery Sticks with Almond Butter

MAKES 1 SERVING

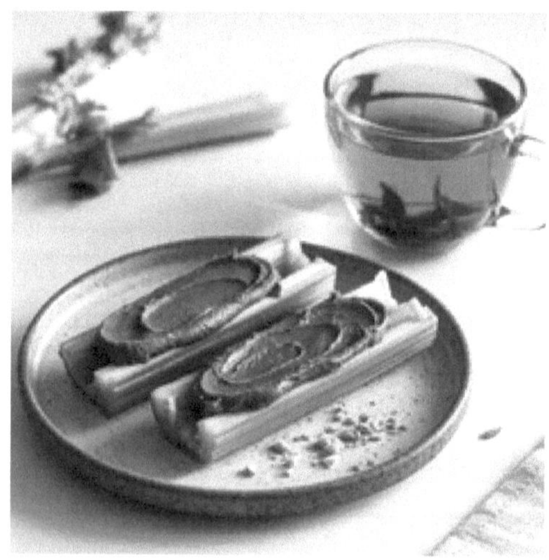

INGREDIENTS:

- 2 celery stalks
- 2 tbsp unsweetened almond butter

DIRECTIONS:

1. Trim celery stalks and cut in half if desired.
2. Spread 1 tbsp almond butter on each stalk.
3. Serve immediately or pack for an on-the-go snack.
4. It's simple, balanced, and great for an afternoon energy lift.

62. Carrots and Celery with Flaxseed and Almond Butter

MAKES 1 SERVING

INGREDIENTS:

- 10 baby carrots
- 2 celery stalks, halved

- 2 tbsp unsweetened almond butter
- 2 tbsp ground flaxseed

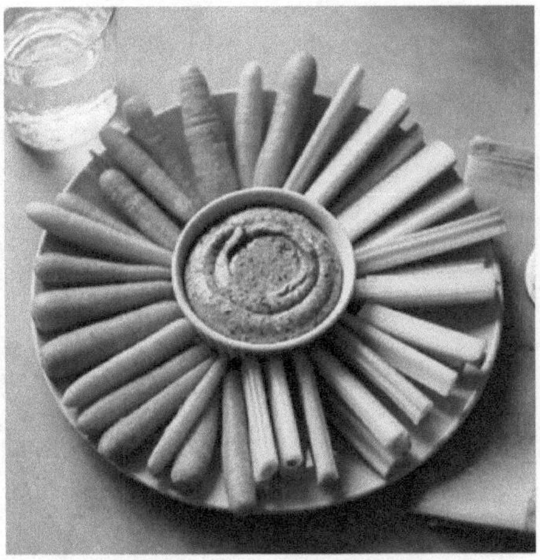

DIRECTIONS:

1. In a small bowl, stir almond butter with flaxseed until smooth.
2. Dip carrots and celery into the mixture.
3. This snack supports hormone detox with fiber and lignans from flax and is ideal for curbing mid-afternoon cravings.

63. Caprese Bites

MAKES 24 MINI SKEWERS (SERVES 4)

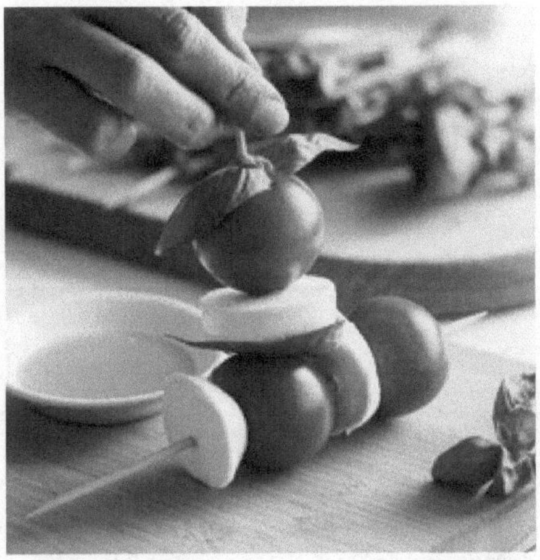

INGREDIENTS:

- 24 cherry tomatoes
- 24 basil leaves
- 8 oz fresh mozzarella balls
- 24 small skewers
- Olive oil

DIRECTIONS:

1. On each skewer, thread 1 tomato, 1 folded basil leaf, and 1 mozzarella ball.
2. Arrange on a platter and drizzle with olive oil just before serving.
3. Serve 3–4 skewers per person for a satisfying snack or appetizer.

64. Apple Clusters

MAKES 1 SERVING

INGREDIENTS:

- 1 small apple, cored and sliced
- 2 tbsp unsweetened almond butter
- 1 tbsp chia seeds
- 1 tbsp ground flaxseed
- 2 tbsp unsweetened coconut flakes

DIRECTIONS:

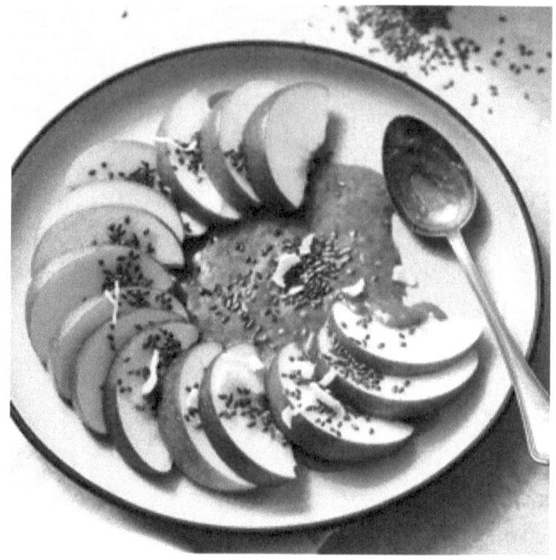

1. Arrange the apple slices in a circle on a plate.
2. In a small microwave-safe bowl, combine almond butter, chia seeds, and flaxseed. Microwave for 15–30 seconds until slightly melted.
3. Drizzle the almond butter mixture over the apple slices.
4. Sprinkle with coconut flakes and enjoy immediately.
5. This snack delivers antioxidants, protein, and omega-3s in every bite.

65. Aloha Avocado

MAKES 4 SERVINGS

INGREDIENTS:

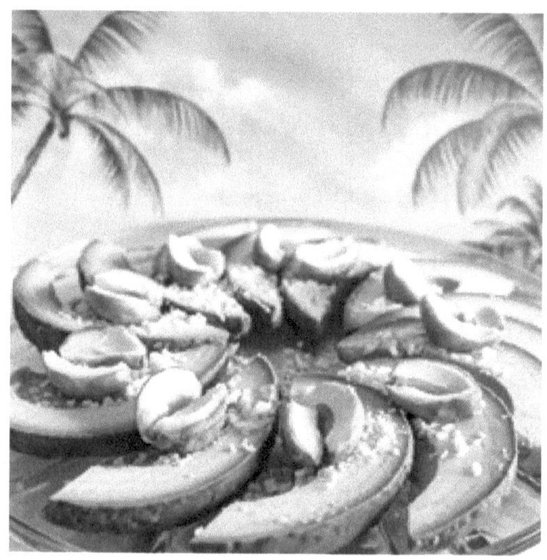

- 2 ripe avocados
- 1 cup halved macadamia nuts
- ½ cup unsweetened coconut flakes

DIRECTIONS:

1. Cut each avocado in half and remove the pits. Slice each half into quarters.
2. Arrange on a platter and sprinkle macadamia nuts into the center of each slice.
3. Finish with a dusting of coconut flakes.
4. Serve immediately or chill for 10 minutes. This low-carb, nutrient-dense snack is great as a post-workout bite or healthy dessert alternative.

66. Pumpkin-Spiced Walnuts

MAKES 1 SERVING

INGREDIENTS:

- ¼ cup whole walnuts
- 1 tsp avocado oil
- ½ tsp pumpkin pie spice

DIRECTIONS:

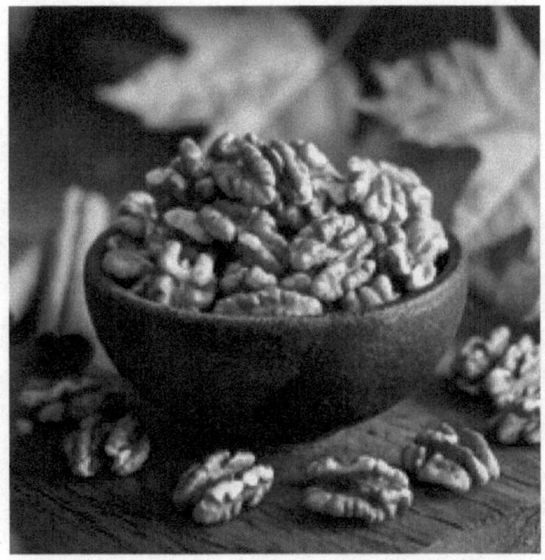

1. Place walnuts in a small bowl. Drizzle with avocado oil and toss to coat evenly.
2. Sprinkle with pumpkin pie spice and stir again.
3. Enjoy immediately or toast for 3–5 minutes in a skillet over low heat to enhance flavor.
4. This snack is rich in omega-3s and perfect for fall, or any time you need a warm, spiced crunch.

67. Avocado Crisps

MAKES 1 SERVING

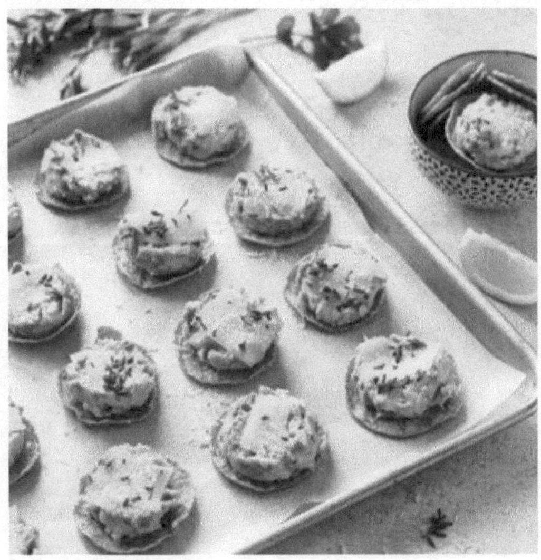

INGREDIENTS:

- 1 ripe avocado, chopped
- ¼ cup grated Parmesan
- 1 tsp lemon juice
- ½ tsp garlic powder
- ½ tsp Italian seasoning

Directions:

1. Preheat oven to 325°F. Line a baking sheet with parchment paper.
2. In a bowl, mash avocado. Stir in Parmesan, lemon juice, garlic powder, and Italian seasoning.
3. Drop teaspoon-sized portions onto baking sheet and flatten.
4. Bake 15–18 minutes, or until edges are browned and crispy.
5. Let cool before eating. These crisps are a great replacement for chips and are high in monounsaturated fats.

68. Cheese and Walnuts

MAKES 1 SERVING

INGREDIENTS:

- ¼ cup walnut halves
- 1 cheese stick (any variety)

DIRECTIONS:

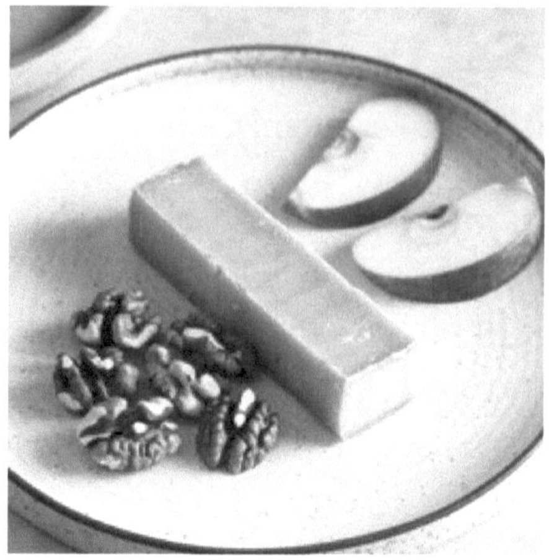

1. Arrange walnut halves on a small plate.

2. Add the cheese stick alongside.

3. Enjoy as is, or pair with a few apple slices for an optional boost of natural sweetness.

4. This pairing delivers protein, calcium, and omega-3s in a portable and convenient format.

69. Herbed White Bean Dip

MAKES 2 SERVINGS (ABOUT ¾ CUP)

INGREDIENTS:

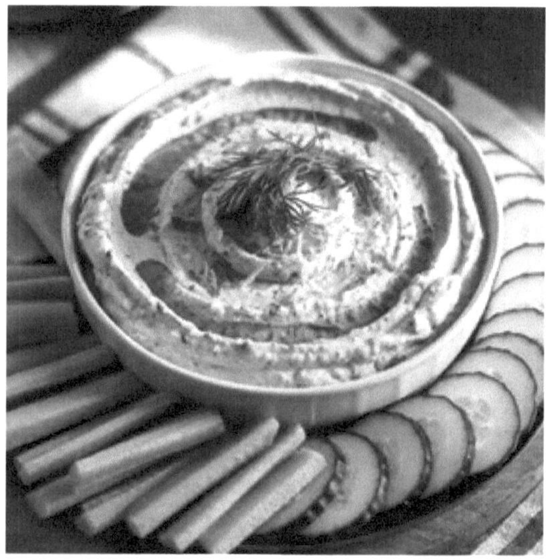

- ½ cup cooked cannellini beans
- ½ lemon, juiced (about 1½ tbsp)
- 1 tsp grated lemon zest
- 2 tbsp tahini or soy sauce
- 1 tbsp olive oil
- 1 tbsp chopped fresh dill
- 1 garlic clove

DIRECTIONS:

1. Add all ingredients to a food processor and blend until smooth.

2. Taste and adjust seasoning as needed.

3. Transfer to a small bowl and serve with cucumbers, carrots, or bell pepper strips.

4. This dip offers plant protein, omega-3s from tahini, and detox-friendly garlic and lemon.

70. Herbed Cottage Cheese Dip with Cucumber

MAKES 2 SERVINGS

INGREDIENTS:

- ½ cup full-fat cottage cheese
- 1 tbsp fresh lemon juice

- ½ tsp garlic powder
- ½ tsp onion powder
- ¼ tsp black pepper
- 1 tbsp chopped fresh dill
- 1 small cucumber, sliced

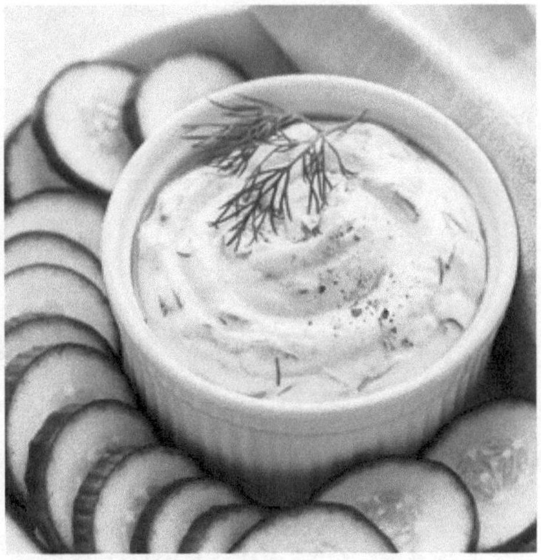

DIRECTIONS:

1. Add cottage cheese, lemon juice, spices, and dill to a blender. Blend until smooth.
2. Transfer to a bowl and serve with cucumber rounds.
3. This refreshing, savory snack is ideal for balancing hunger hormones and supporting muscle maintenance.

71. Veggie Slices with Italian Mayo Dip

MAKES 4 SERVINGS

INGREDIENTS:

- 1 cup olive oil mayonnaise
- 1 tbsp Italian seasoning
- 2 cucumbers, sliced
- 2 large carrots, sliced
- 8 asparagus spears, trimmed and cut
- 8 radishes, halved or quartered

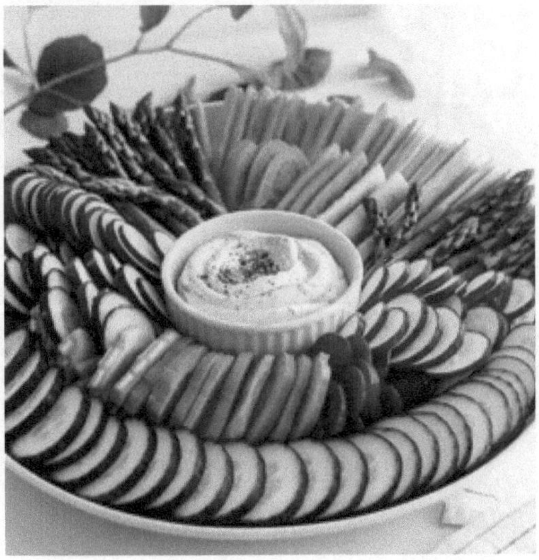

DIRECTIONS:

1. In a small bowl, stir together mayo and Italian seasoning until smooth.
2. Arrange all sliced vegetables on a platter.
3. Serve with the dip for dunking.
4. Perfect for a hormone-balancing snack plate or party-friendly appetizer.

72. Marinated Olives, Chickpeas, and Vegetables with Thyme and Dill

MAKES 4 SERVINGS

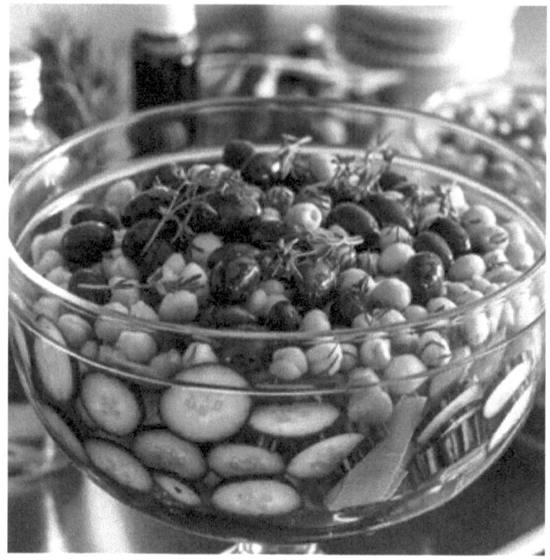

INGREDIENTS:

- 2 cucumbers, sliced
- 2 carrots, sliced
- 1 (15 oz) can chickpeas, rinsed and drained
- 2 cups olives (any kind)
- ½ cup red wine vinegar
- ¼ cup fresh thyme leaves
- ¼ cup fresh dill

DIRECTIONS:

1. Combine cucumbers, carrots, chickpeas, and olives in a large bowl.
2. Add vinegar, thyme, and dill. Stir to coat.
3. Cover and refrigerate for 15 minutes before serving.
4. Eat alone as a protein-rich snack or spoon over greens for a tangy salad boost.

73. Cucumber, Tomato, and Feta Salad

MAKES 1 SERVING

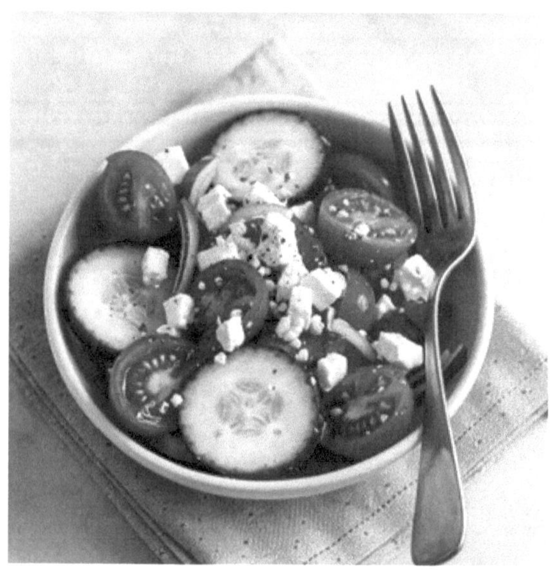

INGREDIENTS:

- 1 medium cucumber, sliced
- 1 cup halved cherry tomatoes
- ¼ small red onion, diced
- 1 garlic clove, minced
- 1 tbsp olive oil
- 1 tbsp red wine vinegar
- 2 tbsp crumbled feta cheese

DIRECTIONS:

1. Combine cucumber, tomatoes, onion, and garlic in a small bowl.
2. Drizzle with olive oil and vinegar, then toss gently.
3. Sprinkle feta on top and serve immediately.

4. This snack is full of water-rich veggies, bone-supportive calcium, and heart-healthy fats.

VI. Smart Snacks: Wraps, Eggs & Light Protein

Supports: Craving control, fatigue reduction, insulin sensitivity, and protein-rich nourishment

74. Cheese and Walnuts

MAKES 1 SERVING

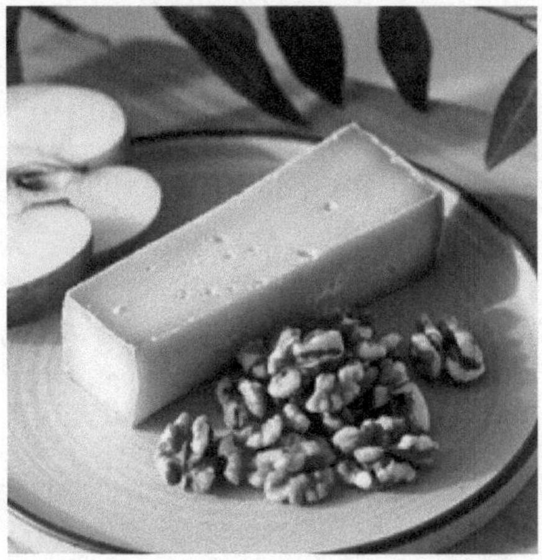

INGREDIENTS:

- ¼ cup walnut halves
- 1 cheese stick (any variety)

DIRECTIONS:

1. Arrange walnut halves on a small plate.
2. Add the cheese stick alongside.
3. Enjoy as is, or pair with a few apple slices for an optional boost of natural sweetness.

75. Herbed Cottage Cheese Dip with Cucumber

MAKES 2 SERVINGS

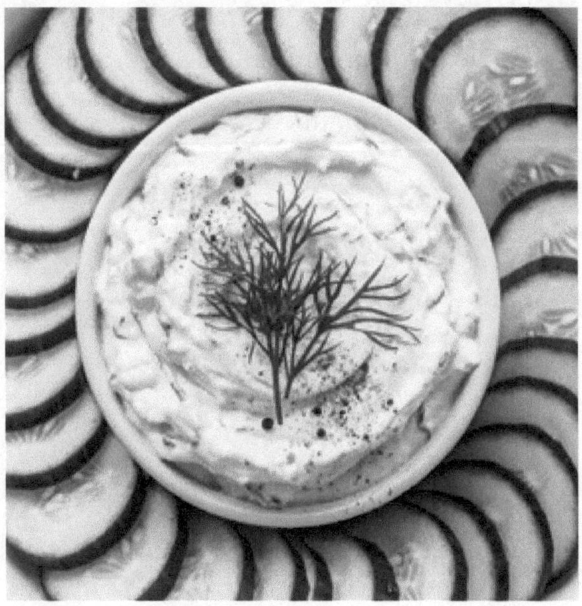

INGREDIENTS:

- ½ cup full-fat cottage cheese
- 1 tbsp fresh lemon juice
- ½ tsp garlic powder
- ½ tsp onion powder
- ¼ tsp black pepper
- 1 tbsp chopped fresh dill
- 1 small cucumber, sliced

DIRECTIONS:

1. Add cottage cheese, lemon juice, garlic powder, onion powder, pepper, and dill to a blender. Blend until creamy and smooth.
2. Transfer to a small bowl and serve with cucumber rounds for dipping.

76. Veggie Slices with Italian Mayo Dip

MAKES 4 SERVINGS

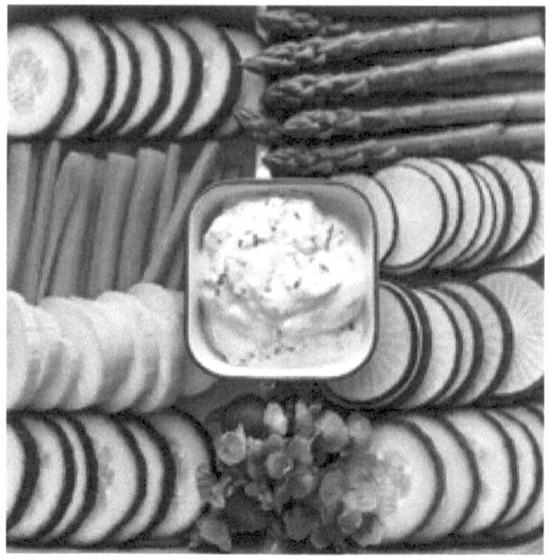

INGREDIENTS:

- 1 cup olive oil mayonnaise
- 1 tbsp Italian seasoning
- 2 cucumbers, sliced
- 2 large carrots, sliced
- 8 asparagus spears, trimmed and halved
- 8 radishes, halved or quartered

DIRECTIONS:

1. In a small bowl, stir together olive oil mayo and Italian seasoning until smooth.
2. Arrange cucumbers, carrots, asparagus, and radishes on a platter or divided snack containers.
3. Serve with mayo dip on the side.

77. Herbed White Bean Dip

MAKES 2 SERVINGS (ABOUT ¾ CUP)

INGREDIENTS:

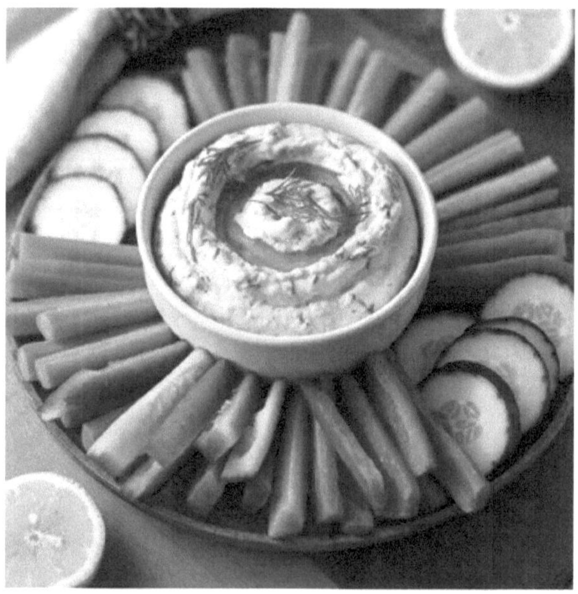

- ½ cup cooked cannellini beans
- 1½ tbsp lemon juice
- 1 tsp grated lemon zest
- 2 tbsp tahini or soy sauce
- 1 tbsp olive oil
- 1 tbsp chopped fresh dill
- 1 garlic clove

DIRECTIONS:

1. Add all ingredients to a food processor and blend until smooth. Scrape down sides as needed.
2. Taste and adjust seasoning.
3. Transfer to a bowl and serve with raw veggie sticks or low-carb crackers.

78. Caprese Bites

MAKES 24 MINI SKEWERS (SERVES 4)

INGREDIENTS:

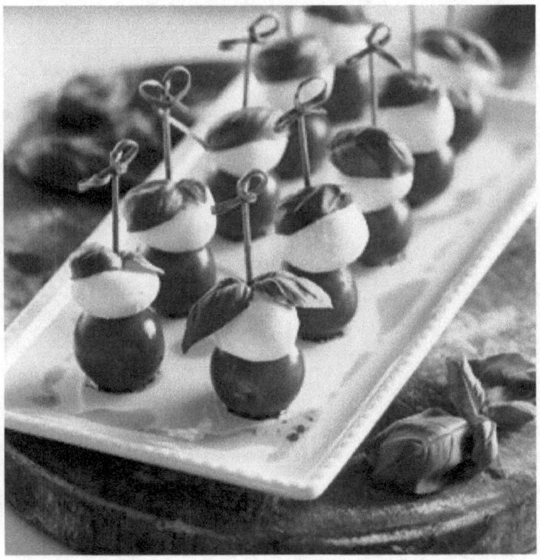

- 24 cherry tomatoes
- 24 fresh basil leaves
- 8 oz fresh mozzarella balls
- 24 small skewers
- Olive oil (for drizzling)

DIRECTIONS:

1. On each skewer, thread 1 cherry tomato, 1 basil leaf (folded), and 1 mozzarella ball.
2. Arrange all skewers on a platter.
3. Just before serving, drizzle with olive oil.

These bites are naturally low-carb, rich in calcium and protein, and full of flavor. Keep a batch ready in the fridge for an easy afternoon snack or elegant appetizer.

79. Turkey and Mayo Lettuce Wraps

MAKES 1 SERVING (2 WRAPS)

INGREDIENTS:

- 1 tbsp olive oil mayonnaise
- 1 tbsp red wine vinegar
- 1 tbsp ground flaxseed
- 2 large lettuce leaves (bibb or romaine)
- 2 oz deli turkey slices
- 1 slice Swiss cheese

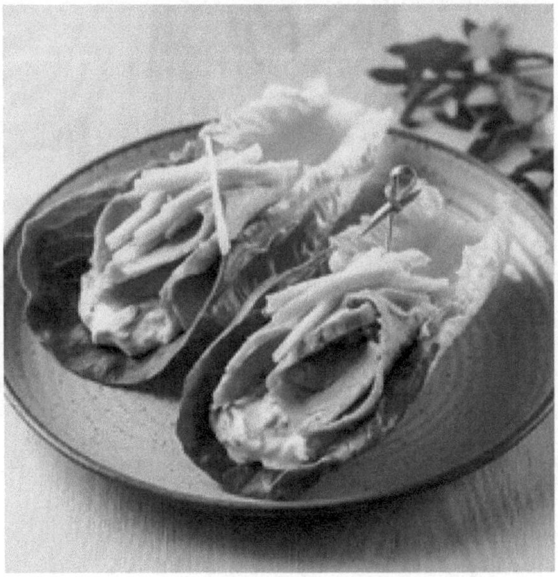

DIRECTIONS:

1. In a small bowl, mix mayonnaise, vinegar, and flaxseed into a spread.
2. Lay lettuce leaves flat and divide the mayo mixture between them.
3. Layer on turkey slices and half a slice of cheese per wrap.

4. Fold and roll to form a hand-held wrap.
5. Enjoy immediately or wrap in parchment for an on-the-go snack.

80. Hard-Boiled Egg with Avocado

MAKES 1 SERVING

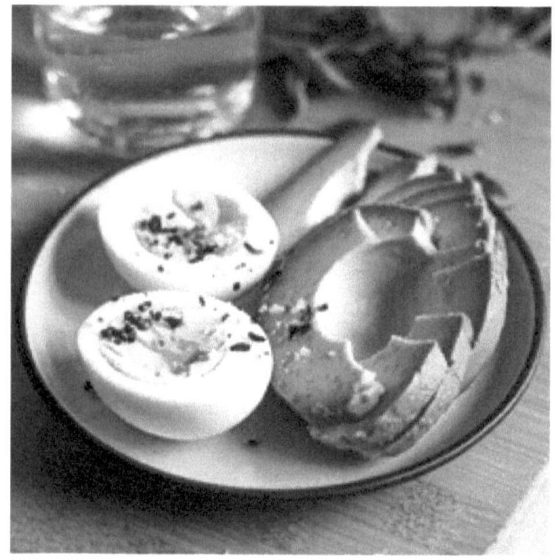

INGREDIENTS:

- 1 hard-boiled egg, peeled and halved
- ½ ripe avocado, sliced

DIRECTIONS:

1. Arrange egg halves and avocado slices on a small plate.
2. Sprinkle with a pinch of sea salt or chili flakes if desired.
3. This snack is perfect post-workout or as a quick pick-me-up in the afternoon.

81. Deviled Eggs with Chia and Turmeric

MAKES 1 SERVING (2 DEVILED EGGS)

INGREDIENTS:

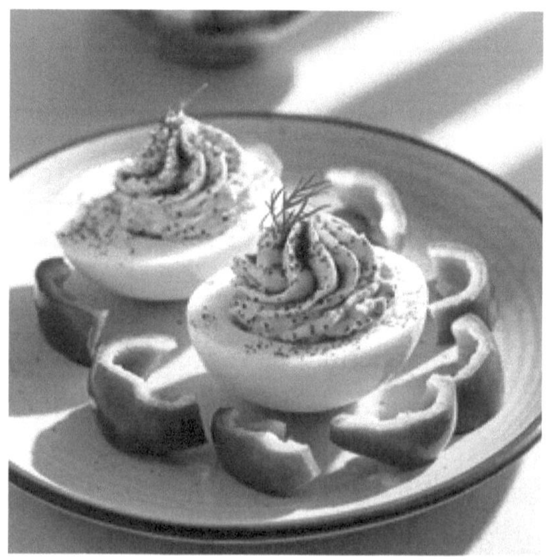

- 2 hard-boiled eggs, halved
- 1 tbsp avocado oil mayo
- 1 tbsp chia seeds
- ¼ tsp ground turmeric
- 1 green bell pepper, sliced (for serving)

DIRECTIONS:

1. Gently scoop yolks into a small bowl and mash with mayo, chia seeds, and turmeric.
2. Spoon filling back into the egg whites.
3. Serve with bell pepper strips for crunch.
4. This snack supports immune health, satiety, and brain function.

82. Naked Turkey Roll-Ups

MAKES 1 SERVING

INGREDIENTS:

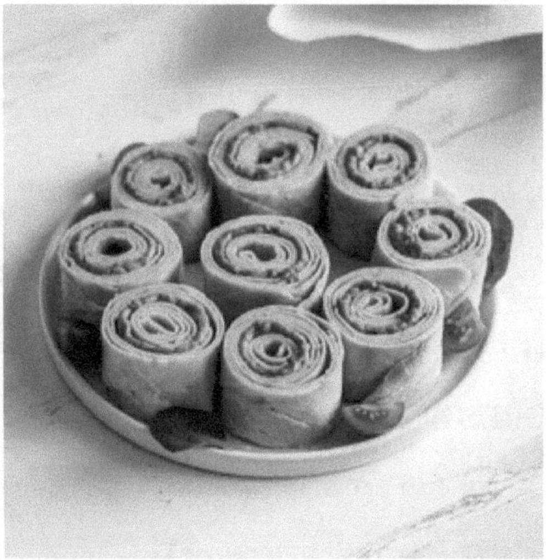

- 2 oz deli turkey slices
- 2 oz Swiss cheese slices
- 1 tbsp spicy brown mustard

DIRECTIONS:

1. Lay turkey slices flat and top each with a slice of cheese.
2. Spread a thin layer of mustard across the top and roll up tightly.
3. Slice in half if desired and enjoy immediately.
4. A great snack with zero prep required and balanced macronutrients.

83. Edamame Mash Salad

MAKES 4 SERVINGS

INGREDIENTS:

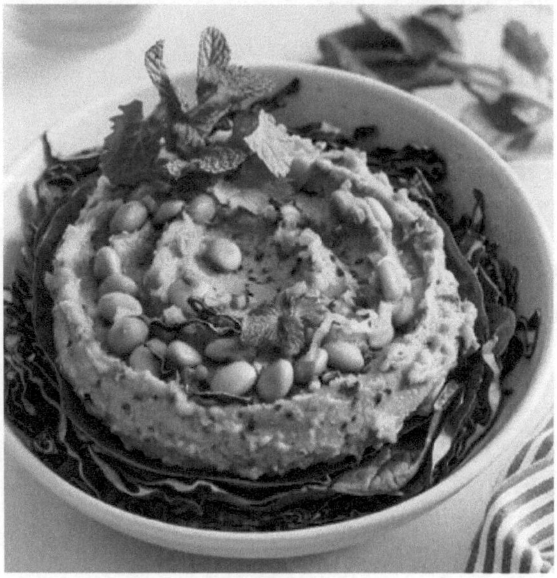

- 1½ cups frozen edamame
- 2 cups boiling water
- 2 garlic cloves
- 1 tbsp lime juice
- 2½ tbsp avocado oil mayo
- 2 tbsp fresh cilantro, minced
- 1 tbsp each minced mint and dill
- ¼ tsp stone-ground mustard
- ¼ tsp salt, ¼ tsp pepper
- 4 cups spinach
- 1 cup shredded red cabbage

DIRECTIONS:

1. Soak edamame in boiling water for 5 minutes, then rinse with cool water.
2. Pulse all mash ingredients in a food processor until blended but textured.

3. Divide spinach and cabbage across 4 bowls. Top with edamame mash and serve.

4. Great for batch prep and ideal for hormone support with phytoestrogens and fiber.

VII. Naturally Sweet Treats & Hormone-Friendly Delights

Supports: Mood lifting, stress relief, sweet satisfaction without sugar crashes, and anti-aging nutrition

84. Pecans with Berries and Coconut

MAKES 1 SERVING

INGREDIENTS:

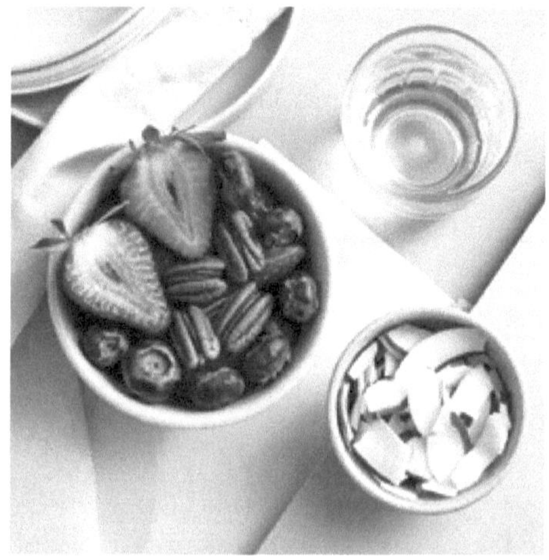

- ¼ cup pecans
- ¼ cup fresh blueberries
- ¼ cup fresh strawberries, sliced
- 2 tbsp unsweetened coconut flakes

DIRECTIONS:

1. Combine all ingredients in a small bowl.
2. Mix gently and enjoy immediately.
3. This simple snack is perfect for satisfying sweet cravings in a nutrient-dense way and makes a great midday refresher.

85. Pecans and Dark Chocolate

MAKES 1 SERVING

INGREDIENTS:

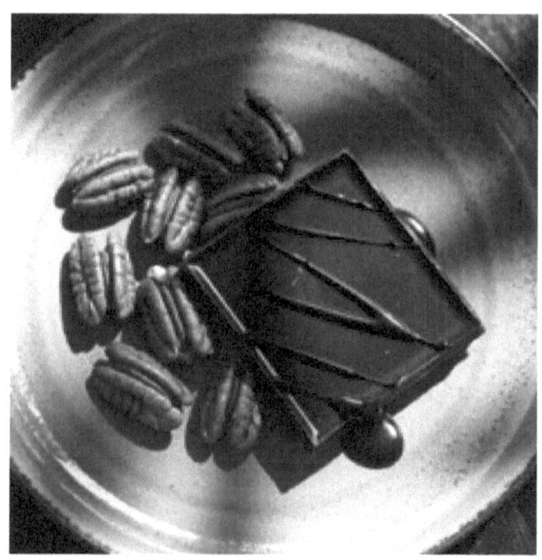

- 1 oz piece of 70% or darker chocolate
- ¼ cup pecans

DIRECTIONS:

1. Enjoy chocolate and pecans together, either side-by-side or with chocolate melted for dipping.
2. For a warm treat, microwave chocolate for 15–20 seconds and drizzle over pecans.
3. This snack delivers hormone-friendly nutrients in a portion-controlled indulgence.

86. Raspberries with Pecans

MAKES 1 SERVING

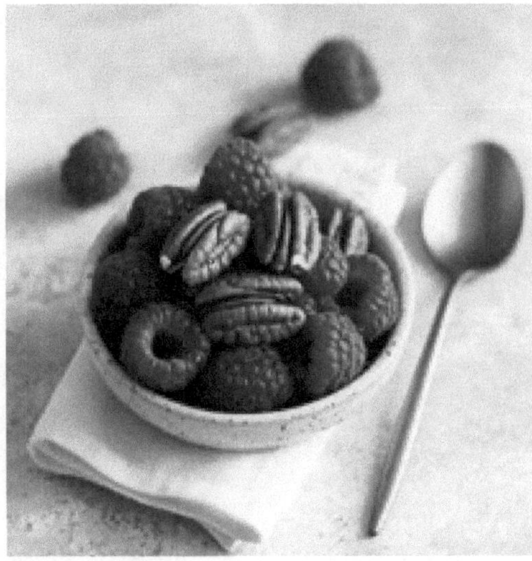

INGREDIENTS:

- ½ cup fresh raspberries
- ¼ cup pecans

DIRECTIONS:

1. Place raspberries and pecans in a small bowl.
2. Eat together with a spoon or finger-food style.
3. This snack is perfect for summer, and pairs well with green tea or a slice of hard cheese if you want to add protein.

87. Nutty Berry Bowl

MAKES 1 SERVING

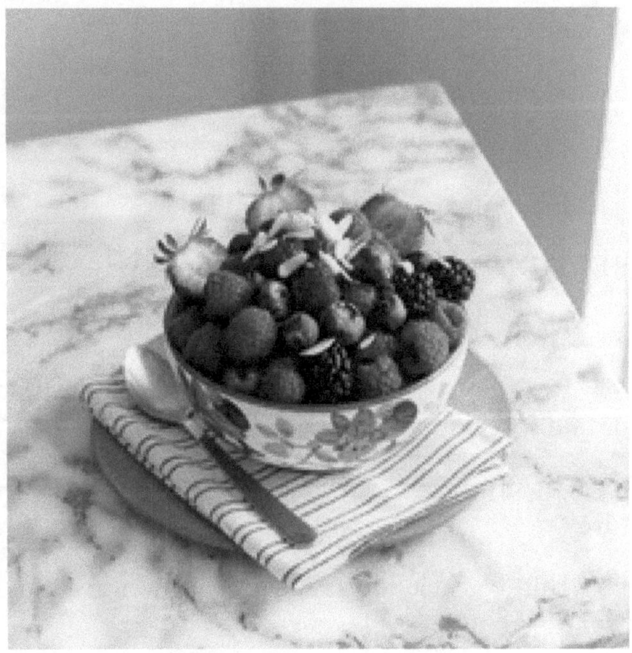

INGREDIENTS:

- ¼ cup strawberries, halved
- ¼ cup raspberries
- ¼ cup blackberries
- ¼ cup blueberries
- 2 tbsp slivered almonds

DIRECTIONS:

1. Combine all berries in a bowl.
2. Top with slivered almonds and serve.
3. Feel free to add chia seeds or Greek yogurt for a more filling version.

88. Tropical Berries

MAKES 1 SERVING

INGREDIENTS:

- ½ cup fresh blueberries
- 2 tbsp unsweetened coconut flakes

DIRECTIONS:

1. Combine blueberries and coconut in a small serving bowl.

2. Toss lightly and enjoy chilled.

3. This naturally sweet combo is anti-inflammatory and supports collagen and gut health.

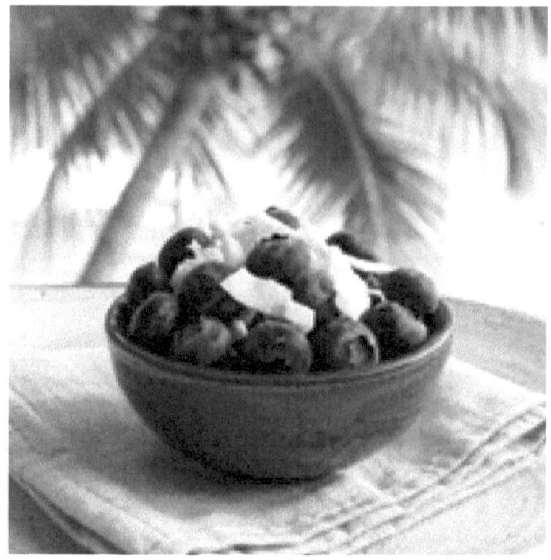

89. Strawberries with Chia Cream

MAKES 1 SERVING

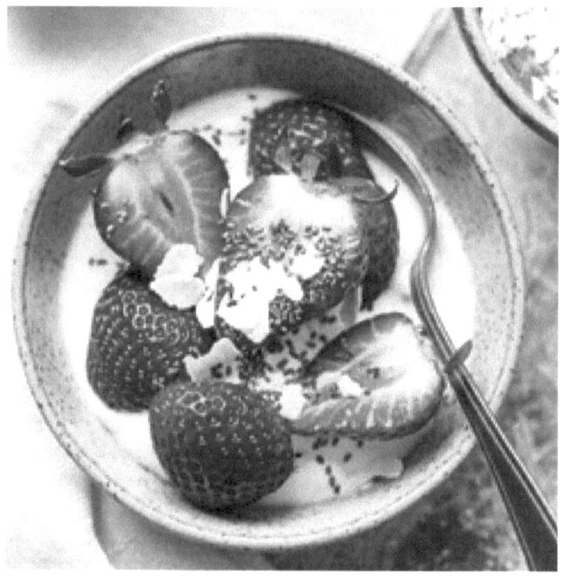

INGREDIENTS:

- 1 cup halved fresh strawberries
- 2 tbsp heavy cream
- 1 tbsp chia seeds
- 1 tbsp unsweetened coconut flakes

DIRECTIONS:

1. Place strawberries in a small bowl.

2. Drizzle with heavy cream, then sprinkle with chia seeds and coconut flakes.

3. Let sit 5 minutes if you prefer a slightly thickened texture.

4. This snack supports satiety and skin health with healthy fats, antioxidants, and collagen-building nutrients.

90. Pear Slices and Ricotta Cheese

MAKES 1 SERVING

INGREDIENTS:

- ½ ripe medium pear, cored and sliced
- ¾ cup whole-milk ricotta (or dairy-free ricotta)
- Dash of ground cinnamon (optional)

DIRECTIONS:

1. Spread pear slices on a plate.
2. Spoon ricotta alongside or on top.
3. Dust with cinnamon if desired.
4. This gentle snack is ideal for quiet mornings, bedtime, or mid-afternoon dips.

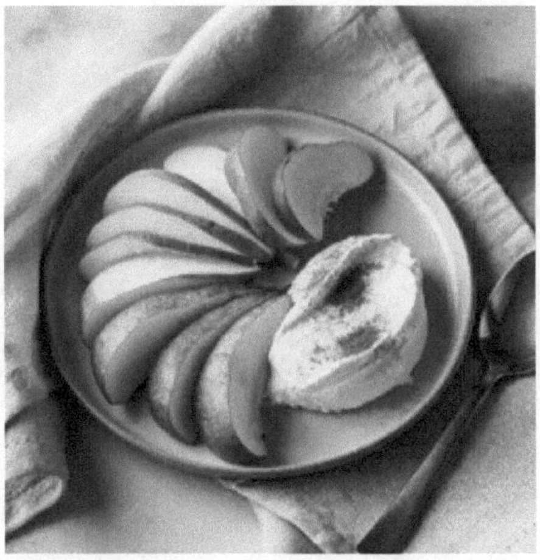

91. Chocolate Mocha Almonds with String Cheese

MAKES 6 SERVINGS

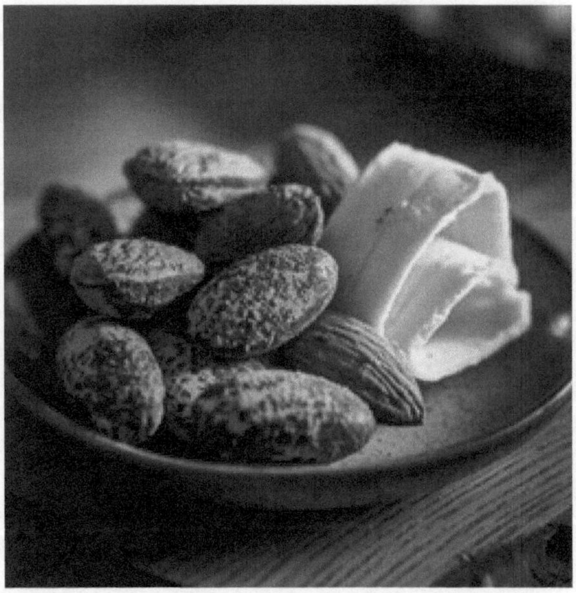

INGREDIENTS:

- 1 cup raw almonds
- ½ tsp olive oil
- 1 tbsp unsweetened cocoa powder
- 1 tsp instant coffee granules
- 1 tsp Swerve or monk fruit sweetener
- 6 string cheeses

DIRECTIONS:

1. Toast almonds in a dry skillet over low heat, stirring often. Drizzle with olive oil.
2. Blend cocoa, coffee, and sweetener. Toss almonds in the mixture and cool.
3. Store almonds in an airtight container. Serve ⅙ of the almonds with 1 string cheese per snack.
4. Rich in healthy fats and protein, this combo curbs cravings and boosts focus.

92. Blueberry Pie Smoothie

MAKES 1 SERVING

INGREDIENTS:

- 2 scoops collagen powder
- 1 scoop MCT powder or 1 tbsp coconut oil

- 1 cup chopped spinach
- ½ cup fresh blueberries
- 2 tbsp chia seeds
- 2 tbsp flaxseed
- 2 tbsp unsweetened almond butter
- ½ tsp almond extract
- Dash of grated nutmeg (optional)

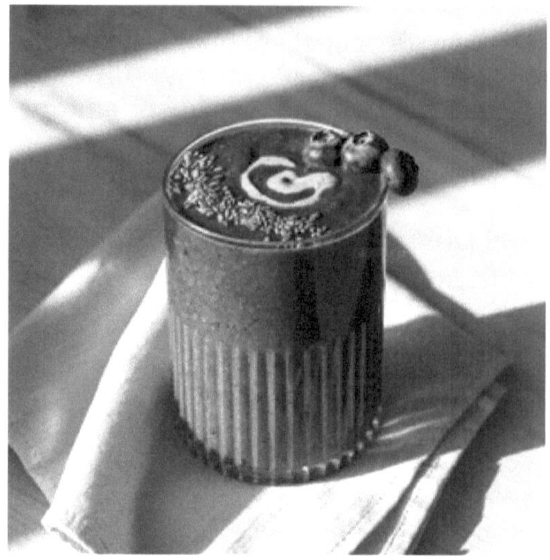

DIRECTIONS:

1. Blend all ingredients until smooth.
2. Pour into a glass and enjoy immediately.
3. Perfect for a hormone-balancing breakfast or recovery shake.

93. Mixed Berry Smoothie

MAKES 1 SERVING

INGREDIENTS:

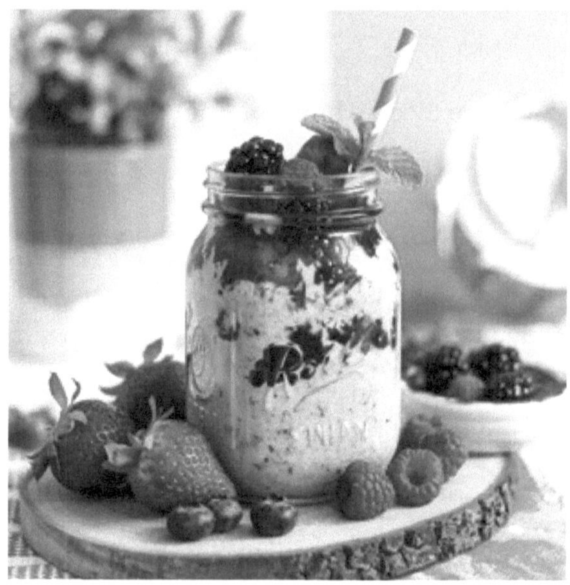

- ¼ cup halved strawberries
- ¼ cup blackberries
- ¼ cup raspberries
- ¼ cup plain full-fat Greek yogurt
- 1 cup baby spinach
- 1 tbsp chia seeds
- 1 tbsp ground flaxseed
- Ice cubes

DIRECTIONS:

1. Add all ingredients to a blender.
2. Blend until smooth. Add water as needed for consistency.
3. This smoothie supports digestion, hormonal balance, and energy throughout the day.

94. Raspberry Almond Smoothie

MAKES 1 SERVING

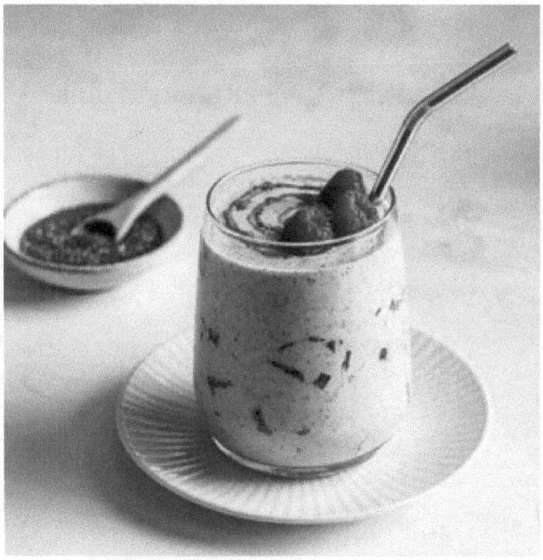

INGREDIENTS:

- ½ cup plain full-fat Greek yogurt
- ½ cup chopped fresh kale
- ¼ cup fresh raspberries
- 1 tbsp unsweetened almond butter
- 1 tbsp chia seeds

DIRECTIONS:

1. Place all ingredients into a high-powered blender.
2. Blend until smooth, adding a splash of water or almond milk to thin if needed.
3. This smoothie is rich in fiber, antioxidants, and healthy fats, great for a quick breakfast or afternoon pick-me-up.

95. Peanut Butter Cup Smoothie

MAKES 1 SERVING

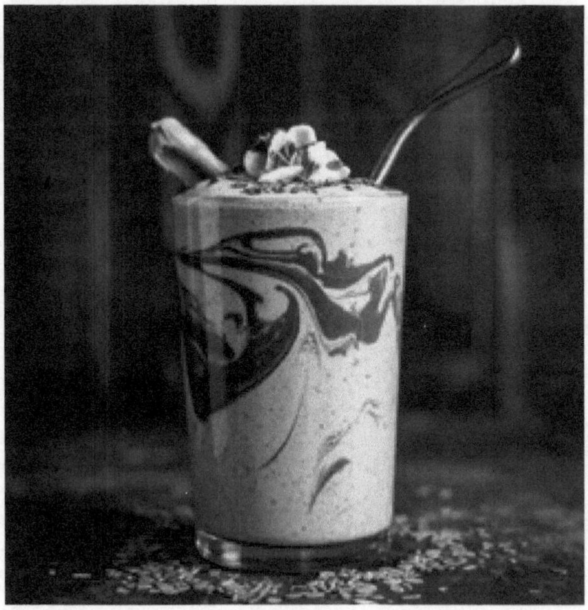

INGREDIENTS:

- ¼ cup plain full-fat Greek yogurt
- 2 tbsp unsweetened cocoa powder
- 2 tbsp no-sugar-added peanut butter
- 1 tbsp ground flaxseed
- ½ tsp vanilla extract
- Ice cubes (optional)

DIRECTIONS:

1. Combine all ingredients in a blender.
2. Blend until creamy and smooth. Add a little water or almond milk to adjust thickness.
3. This treat helps support satiety, muscle repair, and blood sugar stability.

96. Peanut Butter–Mocha Smoothie

MAKES 1 SERVING

INGREDIENTS:

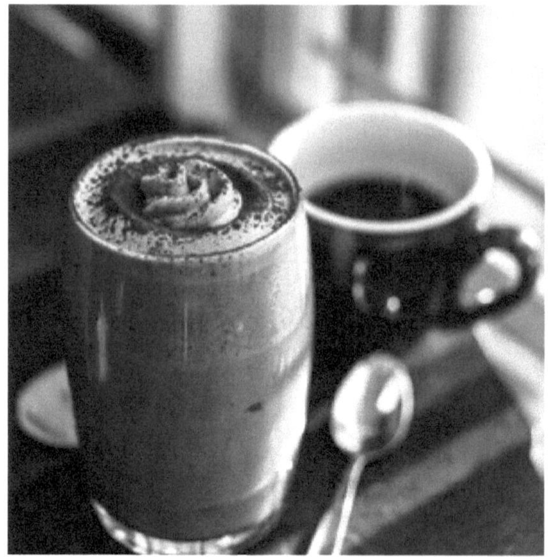

- ½ cup unsweetened almond milk
- 2 tbsp chia seeds
- 2 tbsp ground flaxseed
- 1 tsp unsweetened cocoa powder
- 2 tbsp no-sugar-added peanut butter
- ¼ tsp vanilla extract
- ½ frozen banana
- 1 shot (2 tbsp) espresso
- ⅓ cup crushed ice
- Pinch of salt

DIRECTIONS:

1. Add all ingredients to a blender.
2. Blend on high until smooth and frothy.
3. Enjoy chilled for a protein-rich, caffeinated boost.

97. Green Almond Butter Smoothie

MAKES 1 SERVING

INGREDIENTS:

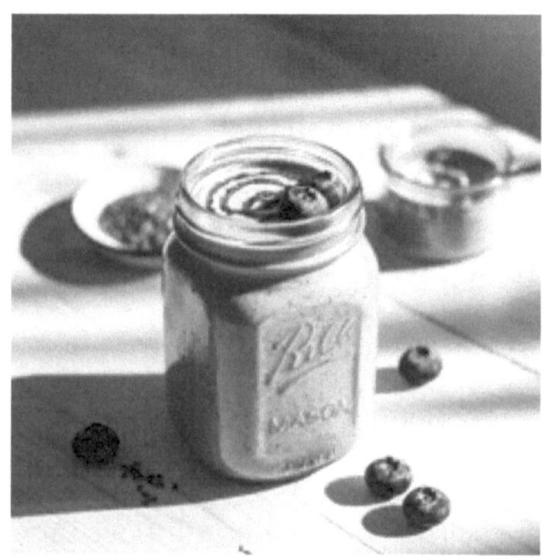

- 1 scoop vegan protein powder
- 1 cup almond milk
- ½ cup fresh blueberries
- 2 tbsp almond butter
- 2 tbsp ground flaxseed

1. Blend all ingredients until smooth.
2. Adjust consistency with more almond milk if needed.
3. This smoothie helps fuel metabolism and muscle repair while balancing blood sugar.

98. Vegan Cinnamon Roll Smoothie

MAKES 1 SERVING

INGREDIENTS:

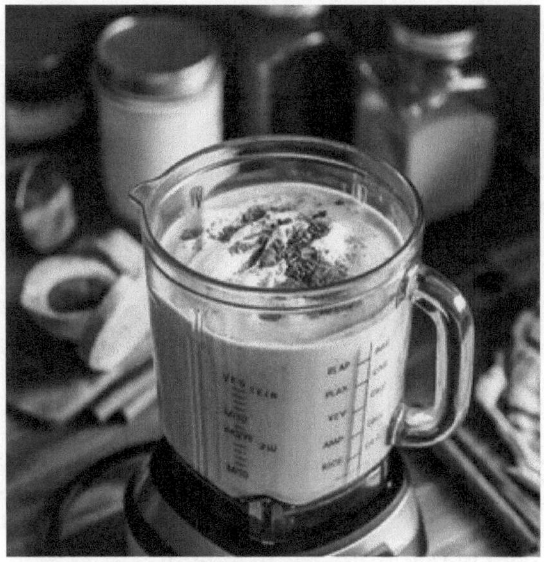

- 2 scoops coconut-based vegan protein powder
- 1 tsp cinnamon
- ½ tsp vanilla extract
- 2 tbsp ground flaxseed
- ¾ cup unsweetened almond milk yogurt
- 1 cup unsweetened almond milk
- 1 cup ice cubes

1. Combine all ingredients in a blender.
2. Blend until smooth and creamy. Serve immediately.
3. Enjoy as a morning meal or post-workout refreshment with anti-inflammatory benefits.

99. Chia Pudding

MAKES 1 SERVING

INGREDIENTS:

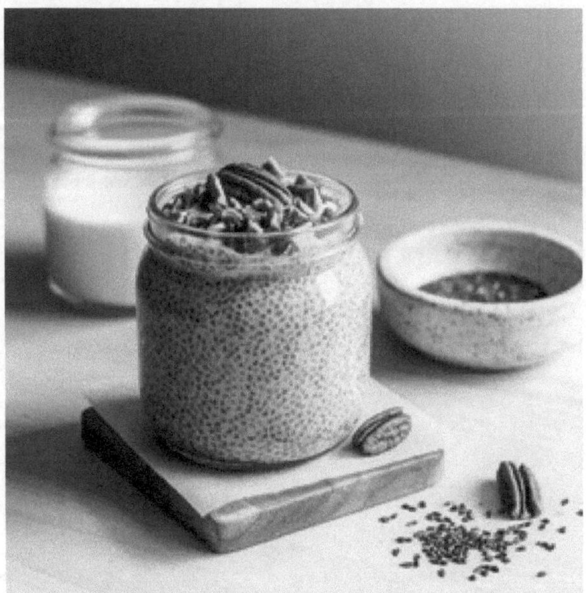

- 1 tbsp flax seeds
- 2 tbsp chopped pecans
- Dash of ground cinnamon
- ½ cup unsweetened coconut milk
- ¼ cup chia seeds

1. In a small bowl, combine flax seeds, pecans, and a sprinkle of cinnamon.
2. Slowly stir in coconut milk to blend evenly.
3. Sprinkle chia seeds on top and stir gently.
4. Cover and refrigerate for at least 4–5 hours, or overnight, until thickened.
5. This creamy, fiber-rich pudding promotes digestion and hormone support while keeping you full for hours.

100. Coconut–Chia Pudding with Raspberries

MAKES 2 SERVINGS

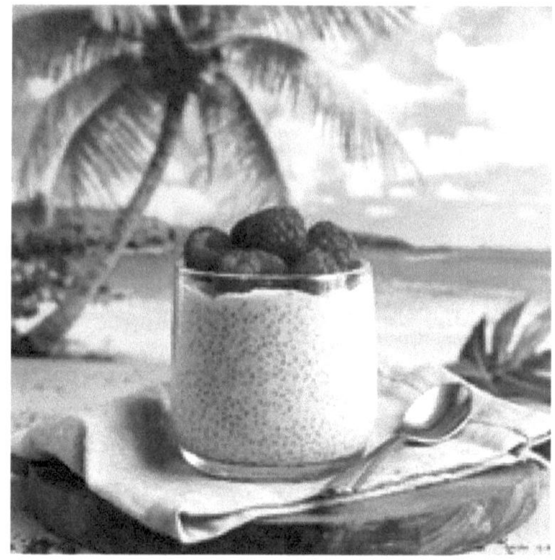

INGREDIENTS:

- 1 (15 oz) can unsweetened coconut milk
- ½ tsp vanilla extract
- Pinch of stevia or monk fruit
- ¼ tsp pumpkin pie spice
- ½ cup chia seeds
- ½ cup fresh raspberries

DIRECTIONS:

1. In a medium bowl, stir together coconut milk, vanilla, sweetener, and spice until smooth.
2. Stir in chia seeds and mix well.
3. Cover and refrigerate for 4+ hours until thickened.
4. Serve topped with fresh raspberries.
5. This pudding is ideal for dessert, a fiber-rich snack, or a morning on-the-go meal.

CHAPTER 10: STAYING BALANCED FOR LIFE

Balance isn't about being perfect. Balance is about having a flexible, sustainable rhythm that nourishes your mind and body even when things get crazy, stressful, or uncertain. The true strength of health isn't in a picture-perfect week of clean food or a faultless morning routine. It's in your capacity to recover, reset, and keep showing up for yourself—over and over.

Let's begin with rhythm. Your body loves routine. Routines on a daily basis with eating, sleeping, exercise, and attitude keep your hormones in check and grounded. By waking and sleeping at about the same time every day, your circadian rhythm becomes stronger. This natural cycle has the ability to keep cortisol, your main stress hormone, in balance. Cortisol is designed to peak in the morning to make you alert and focused. It ought to then gradually decrease during the day, coming to its lowest level in the evening so that you can sleep. When that rhythm gets broken—through chronic stress, inadequate sleep, missed meals, or inflammatory foods—your cortisol can remain elevated during the wrong times. This causes brain fog, weight gain, cravings, lethargy, and anxiety.

One of the best weapons to aid cortisol balance is a regular meal rhythm. You do not have to feed yourself six times a day. Indeed, for most women, consuming two to three nutrient-rich meals in a 10- to 12-hour window is optimal. Add protein, healthy fat, and fiber-rich carbohydrates to every meal to maintain stable blood sugar and avoid crashes that cause irritability and exhaustion. Preventing long periods of fasting followed by binging or emotional eating is also crucial. The objective is not perpetual control—it is consistency. Your body adores feeling certain that nourishment is arriving on a regular and reliable basis.

Physical movement is also a significant contributor to keeping cortisol in check. A short walk after eating can help stabilize blood sugar. Strength training enhances metabolic flexibility and decreases insulin resistance. Yoga, stretching, or just taking five minutes to breathe profoundly allows your nervous system to reset. You don't have to annihilate a workout each day. You do have to move your body with purpose.

For brain fog and low energy, hydration and micronutrients are your best bet. Too often, low energy is mistaken for a lack of motivation when actually it is dehydration or a nutrient deficiency. Begin your day with water and a dash of sea salt. Eat magnesium-rich greens and potassium sources such as avocado and cooked spinach. These help balance electrolytes and stabilize nerve and muscle function. Brain fog can also stem from poor gut health. If you've been inconsistent with fiber or probiotics, gently reintroduce them. Try a tablespoon of ground flaxseed daily, fermented veggies, or a low-sugar probiotic yogurt.

Fatigue is your body's way of whispering that something is out of sync. Sometimes that's sleep. Sometimes it's overexertion. Sometimes it is physical exhaustion or mental overload. One of the most impactful things you can do is check in with yourself truthfully. How am I doing presently? What do I need? Am I attempting to muscle through something that really deserves some attention? Rebalancing isn't always a matter of putting more energy in. Occasionally it's a matter of allowing yourself permission to rest and refocus.

Above all, learn to reboot guilt-free. You are not falling apart when you miss a workout or eat a processed food. You are living. Resilience is not never falling—it's about getting back to what works and not falling into self-judgment. Choose one tiny thing that you can do today. Perhaps it's drinking an entire glass of water before you even have coffee. Perhaps it's adding a protein to your next meal. Perhaps it's shutting your phone off 30 minutes before bedtime. Each of them is a step in the direction of equilibrium.

Your body doesn't want a perfect you. It wants a consistent, loving you. When you discover how to stay in tune with your rhythms, how to recover with care, and how to nurture your body when things go awry, you create lasting confidence. That confidence is not based on discipline or denial—it's based on trust. And that trust is what propels you forward.

SUPPORTING EXTRAS

Conversion Charts

Understanding kitchen measurements can save time and ensure your recipes turn out just right. Use the following charts to help you convert volume, weight, temperature, and international units without guesswork.

Volume Conversions

US Measurement	Equivalent
1 tablespoon	3 teaspoons
¼ cup	4 tablespoons
⅓ cup	5 tablespoons + 1 teaspoon
½ cup	8 tablespoons
1 cup	16 tablespoons
1 fluid ounce (fl oz)	2 tablespoons
1 pint	2 cups
1 quart	4 cups
1 gallon	16 cups

Dry Weight Conversions

Ingredient	1 Cup (approximate)
Almond flour	96 grams
Coconut flour	112 grams
Ground flaxseed	112 grams
Chia seeds	170 grams
Shredded cheese	113 grams
Cooked rice	195 grams
Cauliflower rice	107 grams
Cooked chicken, diced	140 grams

Liquid & Metric Equivalents

US to Metric	
1 cup	240 milliliters (ml)
1 tablespoon	15 ml
1 teaspoon	5 ml
1 fluid ounce	30 ml

Weight Equivalents

1 ounce	28 grams
1 pound	454 grams
Oven Temperature Conversions	
Fahrenheit	Celsius
250°F	120°C
300°F	150°C
325°F	165°C
350°F	175°C
375°F	190°C
400°F	200°C
425°F	220°C
450°F	230°C

Glossary of Terms

Some of the ingredients and terms used in this book may be unfamiliar if you're new to hormone-focused eating. The glossary below will help you understand their roles and benefits in your diet.

Adaptogens

Plant-based compounds that help regulate the body's stress response. Examples include ashwagandha, holy basil, and rhodiola.

Almond flour

A grain-free flour made from finely ground blanched almonds. Common in low-carb and gluten-free baking.

Coconut aminos

A salty, soy sauce alternative made from fermented coconut sap. It's lower in sodium and soy-free.

Chia seeds

Tiny seeds that absorb liquid and form a gel-like texture. High in fiber, omega-3s, and plant-based protein.

Flaxseed (ground)

A source of lignans, fiber, and omega-3 fats. Must be ground for optimal absorption.

Ghee

Clarified butter with the milk solids removed. Often tolerated better than regular butter and used in high-heat cooking.

Glucagon

A hormone that raises blood sugar levels by prompting the liver to release stored glucose.

Glycemic index (GI)

A measure of how quickly a food raises blood sugar. Low-GI foods cause a slower, more stable rise.

Hormone-friendly

Refers to foods and practices that support balanced hormone production, detoxification, and reduced inflammation.

Inflammation

The body's response to injury or stress. Chronic low-grade inflammation is linked to hormonal imbalances and disease.

Macronutrients

The three main nutrient groups: protein, fat, and carbohydrates. Each plays a vital role in energy and hormone regulation.

Metabolism

The set of processes that convert food into energy and regulate bodily functions. Can be influenced by diet, hormones, and muscle mass.

Monk fruit sweetener

A natural, zero-calorie sweetener derived from the monk fruit plant. Often used in low-carb or anti-inflammatory diets.

MCT oil

Short for medium-chain triglycerides, this oil is rapidly absorbed by the body and converted into energy. Found in coconut oil.

Phytoestrogens

Plant-based compounds that can have estrogen-like effects in the body. Found in flaxseed, soy, and legumes.

Resistant starch

A type of carbohydrate that resists digestion and acts like fiber, feeding beneficial gut bacteria.

Satiety

The feeling of fullness and satisfaction after eating. Healthy fats, fiber, and protein all promote satiety.

Seed cycling

A nutritional approach where different seeds are consumed during different phases of the menstrual cycle to support hormone balance.

Spaghetti squash

A low-carb vegetable that naturally forms noodle-like strands when cooked. Often used as a pasta substitute.

Tamari

A gluten-free soy sauce made from fermented soybeans. Slightly thicker and richer in flavor than standard soy sauce.

Zoodles

Spiralized zucchini noodles used in place of traditional pasta. Low in carbs and easy to prepare.

Resource Guide

This guide is a starting point for exploring trustworthy brands, communities, and references that align with the Galveston Diet and anti-inflammatory eating.

Pantry Staples & Product Brands

Primal Kitchen – Sauces, dressings, and mayo made without added sugar or seed oils

Simple Mills – Almond flour crackers and baking mixes with clean ingredients

Chosen Foods – Avocado oils and sprays for high-heat cooking

Nutpods – Unsweetened almond and coconut milk creamers

Bob's Red Mill – Ground flaxseed, chia seeds, almond flour, and coconut flour

Wild Planet – Sustainably caught canned tuna and salmon

Meal Prep Tools & Kitchen Gear

Instant Pot or slow cooker – For batch cooking hormone-friendly soups and stews

Glass storage containers – Ideal for meal prep and avoiding plastic exposure

High-speed blender – For smoothies, chia pudding, and sauces

Spiralizer – Create vegetable noodles like zoodles in minutes

Digital meat thermometer – Helps prevent overcooking lean proteins

Supportive Apps

Carb Manager – For tracking macros and net carbs

MyFitnessPal – Log meals, track nutrients, and view progress

Insight Timer – Guided meditations and stress reduction tools

FastHabit – For intermittent fasting tracking

Yuka – Scan products and get ingredient health scores